INFERTILITY LIES

INFERTILITY LIES

A JOURNEY OF DISCOVERING TRUTH

DR. KAREN SNOW, ND

Infertility Lies: A Journey of Discovering Truth

This book is not intended as a substitute for the medical or psychiatric advice of qualified healthcare professionals. The reader should regularly consult healthcare professionals in matters relating to their health and particularly with respect to any symptoms that may require diagnosis or medical attention.

ISBN: 978-1-7780514-3-2 (paperback)
ISBN: 978-1-7780514-5-6 (hardcover)
ISBN: 978-1-7780514-4-9 (ebook)

Edited by Kate Cooper
Copyedited by Melissa Smith

www.infertilitylies.com

DEDICATION

To my son Pete, to know you is to love you. Our journey to you was worth every moment, our life with you is a dream come true.

To my husband Erik, you are my rock. Our life is an adventure, and I'm so happy it's with you.

Contents

Acknowledgements xi

Introduction

Life is Made up of Seasons 3

Seasons Change 17

Living Through the Storm 25

The Lies

Lie #1: My Plan is the Best Plan 33

Lie #2: Having Children is the Ticket to Happiness 39

Lie #3: The Future is Ours to Control 55

Lie #4: Infertility is a Season of Being Stuck 61

Lie #5: Infertility is a Lone Journey 69

Lie #6: Infertility = Inadequacy 77

Lie #7: Infertility is My Identity 83

Lie #8: Nothing Good can Come from Infertility 91

Lie #9: Success is a Positive Pregnancy Test 101

Lie #10: We Must Always Work Harder 107

Boundaries

Finding Purpose in the Rough Seasons 119

Boundaries with your Time 125

Boundaries for your Treatment 131

Boundaries with Communication 139

Boundaries to Protect your Partner Relationship 149

Final Thoughts

Supporting People through Infertility 159

Acknowledging and Preventing Burnout 167

My Faith and Infertility 179

Seasons Change 189

Your Infertility Legacy 199

About the Author 203
References 205
Resources 209
Connect with Karen 211

ACKNOWLEDGEMENTS

My deepest gratitude to these brilliant women:

Kate Cooper MEd, Sharon Kennie, Amanda Smith CPA, CA, Angie Sutton, Nicole Langman, MSW, author of *You Are Wanted-Reclaiming the Truth of Who You Are*, Toni Nieuwhof, author of *Before You Split,* Em Dyson MSW, Christina Orfanakos MSW, Dr. Erin Wiebe, ND, Dr. Kelly McGuire, ND.

My heartfelt thanks to my sisters and soul-sisters for their unwavering support through this entire journey. I would not be where I am without your love and consistent cheerleading:

Jennifer Hill, Janessa Matta, Jocelyn Whitehead, Karen Giroux, Kendra Penny

To my family and friends, my life is richer with you in it. I've been blessed beyond measure with some of the best people in my circle.

INTRODUCTION

LIFE IS MADE UP OF SEASONS

Life as we know it can change in an instant. A significant life-changing phone call or a collection of small moments can cause our life to look very different than it did just moments earlier. I remember being at the Foo Fighters' *Broken Leg Tour* concert in Toronto one summer evening. My cell phone alarm buzzed at 10 p.m., alerting me to take a hormone injection. Off I went to the public bathroom, tucked myself into a stall, prepared and administered the injection. I was in a season of living my everyday life, layered with intrusive fertility treatment protocols. Some moments change the direction of our lives. The degrees of impact will vary, but we *all* face them. My life had moments that led to change, which felt like a complete change of seasons, where the axis upon which my world was spinning wholly shifted. If you're reading this book, my guess is you've felt your world shift unexpectedly too.

Our personal infertility story has been about loss, growth,

despair, and hope. It's been one of both unfulfilled expectations and immense excitement for a future that's more than we could have imagined. A vast array of emotions have been felt as the dichotomy of this experience unfolded. By processing the feelings of the infertility experience and the full effect of a life-shifting journey, I was encouraged to see the value in learning how to navigate the adventure. There was learning, growth, a deeper awareness of myself, and a newly created outlook on life. It's fascinating how facing challenges allows us to appreciate the capacity of the human spirit to overcome them.

You may find yourself in a place of uncertainty now, feeling overwhelmed by the weight of your own experiences. I discovered that a softening can happen when we view life's challenges in the context of seasons. This time you are living through is a time that will pass – a time that will evolve into a different season as the weather patterns of your life begin to change. You can't control the length of the season or the harrowing experiences that you have been forced to live through. However, seasons inevitably change, weather patterns shift, and day by day, you will see a new season begin to reveal itself.

Even if you feel lonely or isolated, you're not alone in your journey and struggle through infertility – or other challenges life throws your way. Life can feel lonely when you're in the mess of it. Through these words and my story, I hope you know that you are not alone. May you feel validated in your experience and its intense challenges and feel empowered, because it takes a great deal of strength to live through *any* season of pain. Finally, I hope you will come to know and believe in the deepest core of your being that you are valuable, precisely as you are regardless of any outcome, in this current season you are in, and always. Thank you for joining me here.

My Early Story: A Change of Season

Blindly optimistic is how I would describe myself from 1987, when I took my first breath, to 2013, when we were expecting our first child. At this moment, I had not yet felt the change in the winds or noticed the shifting weather patterns; I had not noticed any signs that a change of season was approaching. I was living in the sunshine and enjoying this calm, predictable season of my life. I was a little over a year into my career as a naturopathic doctor. My husband Erik and I had been happily married for three years. Life was rolling along according to plan. After one month of trying to conceive, we were pregnant and could not be more excited. We dressed up our chocolate lab, Buddy, in a "Big Brother" t-shirt and enjoyed sharing our news at my 26th birthday celebration. Both sides of our family were in attendance, excited for the first grandchild on both sides of the family. I was ready to settle into the full-time mom/part-time doctor role as we began to grow our family. Life was good, and things were getting exciting.

If I knew the journey ahead of me at the time, I would never have believed it. Not for me. Things worked out for me, for us. You don't realize how quickly you can attach to a little growing baby until a heartbeat is undetected and you start bleeding a few days later. We miscarried at nine weeks. It took work to maintain our optimism while grieving this life we lost. It was challenging and unexpected.

We dusted ourselves off and anxiously awaited the next positive pregnancy test we were sure was just around the corner, until it wasn't.

A year later, we embarked on our infertility medical treatments. It was a long journey – two natural "timed-intercourse" cycles, six intrauterine inseminations (IUIs), and two rounds of in vitro fertilization (IVF). We were faced with a reality we feared yet never believed would be *our* reality. In fact, years earlier, we had said in a random conversation that we would "never do IVF." I learned many times over, *never say never*. We were diagnosed with unexplained infertility after all the testing and procedures. The smooth waters we once sailed were now a full-on turbulent storm.

This journey has been filled with intensely raw emotion, soul searching, self-discovery, and the complex learning of self-compassion. I did not want to share this part of my story until it was entirely tied off with a beautiful bow, and the result of our efforts was actualized in the form of a growing family. I have since learned that life isn't about the result of whatever situation we are facing, but rather the process and learning that comes with it. Connecting with others through shared experience and being joyful in the hope of what's to come is invaluable when facing life's trials. There is purpose and meaning in hard seasons. The challenges we face in life aren't things to be ashamed of.

These character-defining circumstances, these situations that cause us to evaluate the very core of who we are, what we stand for, and the depths of our resilience, have a purpose. No one is exempt. These challenges aren't based on fair play, nor are they based on whether we feel equipped to manage such a challenge or not. Some seasons carry an intense urgency to end the turmoil and catapult to the other side of the struggle that is only surpassed by the tenacity of the human spirit. The fuel that propels us forward is that part of us that refuses to give up without a fight. In reflecting on my experience, I've fully appreciated the resiliency that needed to be developed throughout this journey.

This book is about my journey through infertility. These lessons surfaced from uncovering several lies I believed to be true that simply weren't. This season held some of the most significant pain in my life. So much pain, so much learning, so much hope. When you view your challenges as opportunities for growth, you open yourself up to the refining process as you become who you are meant to be. We are all in the process of becoming, and we can find purpose in our pain. Acknowledging our innate desire to control our lives that truly cannot be controlled and accepting that learning is an ongoing process will ease the building tension.

In the first few years of infertility, I could not even allow myself to think of my future in any other way than a positive pregnancy test. Now, I can't imagine it any other way than how our life is playing out with our beautiful son, Pete. This experience has been transformative because life is both brutal and beautiful.

While my optimistic personality still shines through, a sprinkling of realism helps keep me grounded and has been a blessing in my life and my work as a naturopathic doctor (ND). Things rarely work out precisely as anyone plans for them to, and sometimes they just don't work out. Being open to plans changing and viewing life as an adventure that is unfolding has proven to be helpful for me. Life is not a structured rubric that we robotically and monotonously track along with. If you've been on this earth for any length of time, you'll intimately know this to be true for you too, I'm sure. Here are my humble insights as an ND turned infertility patient, providing some insight, hope and advice for wherever you are on your journey.

Early Days of Infertility

I grew up on a farm in the small village of Cookstown, Ontario, so I have been around open fields, large farming equipment, and animals my whole life. Some of these early experiences would color the context of my early days of infertility treatments.

Starting cycle monitoring made me feel like a cow. I felt like a cow going to auction when I was lining up outside the ultrasound clinic and waiting for my appointment with the other women. It was dehumanizing that the process of starting a family was whittled down into small, invasive medical steps. There were tasks to push you through to the next step, and the internal anxiety, unknowns, and lack of control were enough to make me want to scream. Everyone in the line was filled with anticipation and anxiety before learning how their ovaries and uterus progressed with whatever treatment they were on that month. It felt degrading, like I was just another person in a long line of insignificant encounters that day. It was the most significant and impactful thing happening in my life at the time, but the process made me feel like a farm animal.

Arriving early to the appointment was imperative to solidify an earlier time slot, as the ultrasound clinic operates on a first-come, first-served basis. The earlier your appointment slot, the less waiting and interfering with your work schedule on the other end of it, which was critical with a full work schedule. It was a "hurry up to wait" type of situation meant to avoid the rush and anxiety of getting to work on time. I tended to place a strong emphasis on my punctuality and efficiency of these appointments to prevent tapping into the emotional overwhelm. The anticipation was intense, and the outcome was entirely outside my control. How was my biological makeup responding to medications, and how would that dictate the upcoming steps? All of this fell within the context of these appointments. It was emotionally exhausting: morning appointments, underlying anxiety, fear and worry throughout the day, while waiting for the call from the clinic to share the results and plan. All the while, I was going about life as though everything was fine; nothing was fine.

My first appointment involved taking this all in, understanding the process, and for the first time in this lonely experience, being surrounded by people going through the same struggle as me. Yet, you could hear a pin drop. No one was speaking, not one word. The intensity was high, near palpable, as we all waited and wondered what was to come of all this. We were filled with the same feelings of uncertainty, fear, anxiety, and shame, yet no one spoke a word.

Most people seemed to handle the silence fine and stayed focused on getting to and from the appointment; however, it didn't make sense or feel natural. I simply could not brush shoulders with women going through the same struggle and not at least acknowledge it somehow. I came to see these early-morning wait times as opportunities to connect with others – this is what makes me feel human and ultimately helped me get through the loneliness of the experience during those early days.

We all knew why we were there in the first place. There was no anonymity; not speaking about it didn't change that. There is a vulnerability in just showing up to these clinics. There is a vulnerability in admitting, acknowledging, and sharing with anyone you are trying and having difficulty getting pregnant. We think that isolation can protect us, but it exacerbates the problem. One morning, I was again in line, not a word being spoken, and I asked the woman next to me how she was doing. She responded with audible relief in her voice that it had been tough; she was doing tests to learn why she couldn't conceive the past year. As the science of acoustics would demonstrate, when someone speaks in a room of no other sounds, all can hear it. The deafening silence was broken. Slowly the conversation built from the two of us to many more women ready to engage. This simple question allowed those interested in engaging to connect and share their stories. It was a relieving and comforting time. We were at different treatment stages, with our own unique experiences, yet all facing infertility. It was freeing and brought a sense of relief to the otherwise uptight, uncertain, stressed-out room. It felt so validating to put words to the personal struggle and share it with people who understood. We empathized, shared fears and frustrations, and we all left a little lighter that day. Moving forward, friendships were built and were a great support.

When a couple is facing infertility, it tends to be a topic that isn't discussed outside the home. At the time, I wasn't comfortable or open to sharing my struggles with close friends or family.

Connecting with others at the clinic felt like a safe option met with understanding and anonymity in my day-to-day life. It was what I needed while processing and understanding my feelings about my infertility before opening up to others. It allowed me to soften the sharp isolation I was beginning to feel and the freedom to share openly without impacting my network and community.

Connecting with others facing a similar struggle allowed me to feel less alone. Not everyone will feel this way, and I know some people who felt quite comfortable sharing with others throughout their whole journey. You may be comfortable in sharing your struggle, or you may want to be more private. There is no right or wrong option, it's important to honor what we need for ourselves at the time.

Infertility can be genuinely lonely if we close in and don't reach out to anyone. Connecting with others at the clinic was life-giving and what I desperately needed at that time in my life. It may also be challenging for those who identify as introverts to reach out and connect with others in social situations like this, and maybe it wouldn't be helpful for everyone. The important part is finding connections in a supportive way for you, wherever you're at. Relationships improve psychological and physical well-being; it's immediately beneficial, and we are wired for it. Bringing a human element to what otherwise felt like a bovine experience was critical for my well-being.

These were the early experiences of what would be a year and a half of attempting to conceive without medical intervention, followed by roughly four years of medical treatments. It was a confusing and draining time with many negative pregnancy tests despite all efforts and energy invested in our hope of building a family.

Maybe you can relate, whether you're at the start of your journey, have experienced loss, or are at a crossroads not knowing how to move forward. I believe and understand that no time is genuinely wasted wherever you are. We can so quickly feel this race against a clock or race to catch up to our expectations on how life plays out. Our circumstances don't define who we are, but they help shape us into a stronger version of ourselves. There is a capacity to grow and find glimpses of joy in the process separate from a specific desired outcome.

With the disorientation of infertility, shaken hopes and dreams, and loosening a tight grip on how we think our life is meant to be, we need to remind ourselves that it doesn't have to play out like this. Life can be tough, and we can still be okay.

Look for the Opportunity: Own Your Story

It's not natural for me to share my inadequacies, challenges, and fears; however, I've come to learn that this is what life is all about – learning and growing and sharing from our experiences to connect with others more deeply.

Authentic connection is the spice of life. While we know that no one's life is exactly as they imagined it would be, there's a difference between understanding that and revealing our shortcomings and challenges. As a society, we can be good at putting our best foot forward, sharing the curated and shiny pieces of life ... I know I can too. It's too easy to do in the days of filters and highlight reels.

Are you ever really inspired by those picture-perfect people? Sure, maybe there is a little jealousy to start, a cheap form of inspiration to have it all together as they appear to. As it turns out, I am most inspired by people who dare to be honest about their struggles and the process of working through and overcoming them. The people we are closest to are the people we can be our most authentic selves around. Over the past decade of practice, I've sat across from thousands of people, listening to their stories. Many look like they've got it all together – like, *really* together. Matching outfits, nails done, fit as a whip. You know what, though? They don't! None of us do. And if we ever do, it won't be for long, so take a breather and prepare for the next time life shifts again.

So here I am, consciously choosing connection by sharing my authentic struggles in the hope of supporting others who are walking this shared road.

You are not alone; you don't have to live this season as though you are. Even though the challenges of infertility make you *feel* like you are alone, your feelings are not based on facts here. There is a massive club, one that you never chose to sign up for and don't want to be a part of. Yet here you are, an active member. It is a time you may not feel entirely understood by those around you. You may not feel understood by your partner. At times, you may not even understand yourself. You are understood by many women who have walked this same road of infertility. Don't take your lonely feelings at face value.

Learning and personal growth don't favor life's smooth and easy seasons. We so desperately crave the smooth, and we need them for a reprieve, a breather, and to synthesize the lessons of the unchartered waters. It's in times when life goes off course, in life's unplanned and the unexpected, that we find the most significant growth. In these times, we must dig deep and recalibrate, shift gears from a life that we may have spent years imagining how it would all play out with every little detail. And those details were so perfect, right? Like, if only we could control all of those perfect details, it was all going to work out exactly as it was meant to, right? Wrong. That is simply not life as we know it, and thankfully so, in many cases. These shifts in plans are where the soul-finding and heart-shaping take place. There is grief in mourning the loss of the life we had imagined.

It turns out the hard stuff is the juicy center. You can't tell by observing it or simply standing by. You must sink your teeth into it, and you've got the grit to move through it. Though you likely won't feel like you do right now, your incredible track record for overcoming difficult days has allowed you to be where you are right now. Still standing. Still fighting. You must still put one tired foot in front of the other as your mind and heart battle it out.

My challenge to you in your current season is to open your heart to accept the learning ahead and open your mind to receive the growth made possible only by this same challenge you are facing.

I suspect you and I have something in common. You're reading this book; you find value in being teachable. You're engaging in the active process of staying open to learning what life has for you, particularly during life's challenges. May we always stay open to possibilities, even those not immediately apparent. May we remain teachable and aware of the many lessons to be learned along this wild ride of life.

Suggestions while reading this book:

- Take time to journal your thoughts and feelings along the way to stay connected to your feelings and your own experience as you navigate infertility; there is an opportunity in journaling your journey. According to Baikie and Wilhelm[1], journaling has been shown to help boost your mood, enhance your sense of well-being, reduce symptoms of depression before an important event (think IVF), and improve working memory.

- Answer the guided questions at the end of each chapter to help support your infertility experience and process the content of this book through your lens.

- Ask a close friend or partner to help answer questions if you have difficulty answering for yourself, or simply open dialogue on topics that resonate with you.

- Emotionally tumultuous times are a lot to manage. Remain gentle and non-judgemental with yourself. Offer yourself unlimited self-compassion. Whatever you are feeling is okay – you are facing incredible stress and doing your best.

- You likely aren't in the headspace to cheer for yourself right now, but know that I'm cheering for you.

SEASONS CHANGE

Infertility is a disorienting experience. I felt the winds changing, the world shifting, and the calm weather patterns making way for more volatile skies overhead. My life became unbalanced as a developing urgency to get my bearings took hold. I felt the need to assert control wherever I could in this new period of my life that was beginning to look very different from where I had been and where I desperately wanted to be. Infertility shook me. I felt trapped in an agitated snow globe with my intentions, hopes and dreams left swirling around like snowflakes. In time, with patience, acceptance, and hope, things settled back into order. While in this very stormy "snow globe" disruption, despite my best efforts, I couldn't force everything to settle fast enough. I couldn't control the weather. Everything had to whirl around, travel the unpredictable path, and find its way, in its own time, to where it was meant to be. A lack of power is excruciating. We work so hard to avoid it at all costs, yet it can indeed be the start of a significant change.

Whether you feel your world is just starting to shift, or you are right in the midst of upheaval and chaos, there is hope and purpose in your current struggle. You're in the swirling middle of it, developing resilience. This is a time to hold on to hope. Hang on; you can do this. You have value and meaning, and your story isn't finished yet.

You might be thinking, "That all sounds great, but it's impossible right now."

It's not that easy to just decide to be okay with this new reality. That's true. That is absolutely true. It takes a lot of deliberate work, a careful look inward, and regular self-reflection along the way, not to mention a slew of uncomfortable thoughts and emotions to process. There was a long time when I wasn't okay with where I was in life either. Like, really not okay. My motivation for writing this book came from a lack of emotional support, support that I wish I had to make the journey a little lighter.

As a child, I remember my mom teaching me that "life isn't fair." I wanted everything to be fair because it makes better sense that way. Why couldn't it be fair? The sooner we come to terms with this reality, the easier it is to release our grip on the tendency towards comparison and constantly keep tabs on what's fair and unfair. You're currently on the receiving end of an unfair situation. You didn't choose it, you didn't plan for it, and you're likely feeling unprepared to handle it. It's tough, I get it. Unfortunately, this idealized way of thinking that everything is distributed evenly or everyone gets a fair turn remains a thread in my network of thinking, requiring frequent challenges. Of course, life isn't fair – the injustices are vast and overwhelming, infertility being one of them.

In addition to the frustrating reality that life isn't fair, infertility revealed the hard lesson that working harder doesn't always lead you to the result you are pushing towards. Working hard towards a goal is a great thing to do. As an overachiever by nature, I felt like I had a lifetime of evidence to support the notion that I would be able to outwit an unfair world through careful planning, dedication, and perseverance to achieve that positive pregnancy test. In Grade 4, the start of elementary school sports teams, I was on the smaller and weaker side of the classroom and underdeveloped compared to my teammates. I found myself at the end of the bench of my basketball team. It was the first time I remember acknowledging how I stacked up against my teammates, and it was not well. That summer, I committed to practicing basketball in our shop on the farm. Playing basketball in the shop required thorough sweeping to clear the area of dirt from tractors driving in and out. I've never been afraid of extra work. I started practicing my ball handling and shooting skills to be better and stronger the next year. The following summer, I went with a friend to a local basketball camp called *Thunderhoops*; there, I continued honing my skills, working my way up to the starting line-up of the Cookstown Cougars basketball team.

I understand these are some *tremendous* achievements. If you think this is a story about my great basketball career, it isn't. I didn't make the high school team and did not go on to the WNBA. However, working harder to achieve the desired result stuck with me. For both track and field and cross-country running seasons, I would start training by running along paths in the fields on our farm in advance of the season to be in shape for competition time.

Hard work would generally pay off. I'd study hard and prepare for tests to get the results that I'd set out to achieve. It was a clear effort resulting in a reward that would play out. Hard work, pushing limits, setting goals and launching into action plans was the name of the game. Infertility is not this same game. In fact, it's very different. Working harder is not the determining factor of the outcome.

This idea that we need to work harder links to the belief that something wrong with you can be fixed with careful planning and hard work. This realization that no amount of effort would provide a specific outcome allowed me to see the situation for what it was, and it made space for grief and acceptance of what is.

I was completely caught off guard when infertility struck; this new "challenge" blindsided me.

This was one of the first times I came up against a significant inconsistency between working hard and achieving my goal. I don't mean for this to sound prideful. If anything, it's embarrassing that I was so naive for such a long time. There was no amount of work that would force this process to change course. *No amount of work.* Though that didn't stop me from working. Feelings of inadequacy, frustration, shame, and fear started to grow as the efforts continued, and the results didn't change. This was my central pain point in this journey. It felt incredibly challenging and contradicted how I had otherwise identified with myself. When there was a problem, I would strategize and struggle to develop a solution when needed. So naturally, this did not compute with me, and maybe you're having a hard time coming to terms with this yourself. I needed to offer myself the space to grieve and accept what was.

Our minds are wired to see barriers requiring a different plan, not a complete roadblock. This consistent mindset proves to be a challenge for many of my patients going through infertility. *We expect results when we put in the effort,* whether an "achiever" by nature or not. Maybe we're measuring achievement with the wrong measuring tape. Maybe there is more to this life than simply checking off one task and moving on to the next. Perhaps roadblocks are a way to re-direct, reorient, or re-set.

It was difficult to accept that my level of effort would not directly affect the outcome of this journey. The amount of work being put in, the emotional investment, and the financial expenditure would not translate with certainty into a pregnancy. I found myself traveling to appointments I didn't want to go to, meeting professionals I didn't want to (have to) meet, and subjecting myself to treatments I didn't want to do, which were among the early challenges of infertility. While in an emotionally charged, overwhelmed haze, I invested so much time, energy and resources into a dream without realizing what was ahead or acknowledging that it was my reality and not some altered state of existence.

This is not a dramatized version; infertility rocked my world, and it may be rocking your world too.

My personality, socialization and profession contributed to my personal experience, just like your unique makeup and characteristics will influence your story and experience. As an ND, I'm in the occupation of helping people, so it was difficult to seek help and admit that I was the one who needed it.

I recently read a book on enneagram personality typing called *The Road Back to You*[20] by Ian Morgan Cron and Suzanne Stabile, which was incredibly clarifying. It was validating to learn that my personality type is the "saddest of all personality types when in a situation of not being able to achieve."[20] Somewhere along the way, it wasn't even about having a biological child but about achieving a goal that I was working so hard towards.

It is so clear that I needed this experience to shape and mold me to help me understand myself and others better. Showing up when the outcome remains out of our control is where the real work comes in. It's pretty vulnerable, isn't it?

I can remember meeting with my reproductive endocrinologist to wrap up what I thought was the end of the road for medical treatments after my first round of IVF. A friend of mine had traveled to the city with me for moral support. The meeting was set to discuss what had transpired to make sense of our four failed frozen embryo transfers from that IVF round and to find some closure. After the discussion, our doctor strongly recommended that we move forward with another round of IVF based on the information we had at the time. I felt torn. I was ready to be done with the tormenting life of IVF. I wanted to shut the door and move on. I felt scared. To start another round would mean entering another season of unknown and uncertainty. Yet there was a glimmer of hope that continued. Moving forward with another round of IVF was the epitome of vulnerability at this time – pursuing something with such passion and heart when the outcome can't be known. No amount of work or dedication would change the outcome, yet continuous effort was required to move towards building our family. I needed these gut-wrenching lessons.

I surveyed nearly 50 women who have or are going through the experience of infertility. I asked what some of the greatest struggles were for them. There were many themes among the responses.

They were feeling isolated and alone, feeling like they were the only ones facing this struggle. The *depth of the emotional toll*, with the many ups and downs, heartache, jealousy, anger, the waiting, the hoping and despair, were all exhausting and overwhelming. Falling victim to *"Why me?"* and feeling like their body was "broken." *Lack of control* over outcomes despite controlling many factors such as meticulous treatments, modifying diet and lifestyle, and investing so much into the process.

One participant clearly said: "Just the sheer weight of it all. Wanting something so bad and so deeply that it feels like an inherent gift and natural 'right' in life, and not being able to attain, achieve or force it – literally no matter what you do, no matter how hard you try. I feel that the experience has affected me emotionally, physically and spiritually, and it has stretched me further than I ever thought possible." Can you relate? I know I certainly can. This experience has an emotional weight that isn't always acknowledged or given the time and space it needs to process.

Life's seasons can change when you least expect them, and you can learn to adjust to the new weather patterns. Life can feel totally out of control, and you can still ground yourself in what you know to be true. Your desired outcome or goal can be entirely out of reach while your value and worth remain steadfast and unwavering. Our value and worth as human beings are not rooted in our productivity, achievements, or fertility. Regardless of your fertility journey outcome, your worth does not change. You are valuable.

As an infertile ND, I have come out to the other end of this unexpected journey and am living to tell the tale. You will have a unique story too. We have the scars and battle wounds to prove it, but let's feel proud of where we land. Infertility is a storm. Icy roads. White-out conditions. Hail crashing down. Storm. Grip the wheel and decelerate. Let's move forward together.

LIVING THROUGH THE STORM

I felt the shift in seasons, and there began a very slow acceptance and recognition that this was my new reality.

I was infertile.

Treatments were necessary, and the outcome was uncertain. Understanding the thoughts and feelings that surfaced while navigating this rough and painful time helped make this experience's elements clearer. Words like challenge, struggle, pain, loss, waiting, and inadequacy dominated my self-talk. The initial storm of infertility unfolded a deeper understanding of the pain this new season brought to my life. I realized that the story I was telling myself about my own experience was littered with several false thoughts I had come to believe as truth. These deceitful thoughts did nothing to relieve any pain; instead, they contributed to the pain and discontentment. These lies that the experience of infertility led me to believe simply were not true.

The following series of lies are outlined in the coming pages. Working through their truths took time. Some of them became clear after moving past infertility altogether, and their clarifying thoughts did not come into focus until I was well on the other side of it all. I hope this book provides you with support in your season of uncertainty. Our stories are undoubtedly different, as no two are ever the same. There is beauty in finding meaning and connection in the similarities and common threads of another's experience. May you find a piece of your experience in mine and know you aren't alone, and develop a deeper understanding of what makes your experience unique to you and the lessons that they may bring.

Both personally and professionally, I've learned the impact of how thoughts directly impact feelings. Bringing awareness to these negative thought patterns allowed me to identify the lies I was telling myself. When our thoughts get the best of us and we let them run wild, it's too easy to start believing them to be true. When we believe them to be accurate, our feelings can take over and cause overwhelming discomfort. Our thoughts influence our emotions, and they can also be a window into our underlying feelings that may need to be addressed.

Thoughts can be deceiving – sometimes outright lies – made worse when fueled by uncertainty. I often tell my stressed and anxious patients that we simply cannot believe everything we think; I needed to take my advice at this time.

I found it helpful to take some time to analyze my thoughts and question some of the common messages in my mind, as seen in the examples below. Critically analyzing our inner conversations can be a powerful way to change what we are thinking and telling ourselves, ultimately shifting how we feel and live our lives. It took time to realize that I had unhealthy thought patterns that were going on in my mind, and these thoughts certainly impacted how I felt about myself and how I behaved in my world at the time.

I have learned that my natural tendency is to outwit and outsmart my feelings. It's hard for me to sit with my big feelings for very long. This strategy below was beneficial for me at the time. However, you may find that it isn't specifically helpful for you right now. And that's okay. If that's the case, feel free to skip ahead and jump into the next section. This isn't a strategy to bypass our feelings, although looking back, I can see that I tried to do this very thing. Taking the time to honor our emotions amid a struggle is validating and required to move through them. Being in distress interrupts our ability to access our prefrontal cortex with logical thinking, so explicitly focusing on the analytical aspects of the situation can cause a more spiraling thought process. Our thoughts can be a symptom, a window into our feelings. We can lean into our feelings using our thoughts. These are tools to support the emotional processing of our experience.

I've learned that there is a compelling dance between feeling and thinking; I hope you can find that rhythm for yourself to the tune that works for you. Lean into your emotions and know-how to lean out of them as well. It's not an all-or-nothing experience. Take what is relevant and supportive for you while honoring the complexity and individuality of this experience. While I've learned I can "out-logic" my feelings to avoid the difficulty and discomfort, I have learned the importance of the uncomfortable. It's okay to feel uncomfortable.

It took a long time to realize these were some of the thoughts I was having. They weren't at the surface of my mind, but they did run deep and had a tremendous impact. They contained so much emotion but so little truth. The list of lies was long. Taking the time to reflect on and decode these lies was critical to my healing. No wonder I felt insecure, inadequate, and anxious during this season. I had no control over an outcome that held my confidence and self-worth. This was shaky ground, wildly inaccurate, and a dangerously unhealthy mindset. It felt awful. Can you relate?

The lies you're telling yourself may not be precisely the ones I was telling myself, but I bet they're just as impactful. Pay attention to what you're saying to yourself; it can be insightful, and early intervention of harmful thought patterns can help change the trajectory of an experience.

Our cognitive function and reasoning skills decline when our nervous systems are hijacked by stress. Our amygdala, the part of our brain that is active under stress, alerts our body to a threat, so we are ready to take action. Also known as our fight, flight, or freeze response, this physiological response can help us understand how we behave during stress when we look back from a calm place and wonder why we acted in specific ways. When you are having trouble calming your nervous system down in times of acute stress, it can be helpful to connect with yourself and find ways to soothe your nervous system. This is a normal stress response. Offering yourself compassion during this challenging and stimulating experience can be helpful. Our mind and body are intimately connected. Perhaps reconnect the two by going for a walk in nature, drinking a cup of tea, calling a friend, listening to calming music, taking a bath, or focusing on your breathing by taking slow, controlled breaths. These are just a few ways to tell your body that you are safe, a way to slowly bring your logical reasoning back and calm the overactive nervous system response.

The beauty of time, personal growth, and self-awareness is identifying the thoughts we are telling ourselves, challenging the validity of these thoughts, and changing our perspective to one based on truth. The key is challenging these negative thoughts:

- Is this thought true?

- Is this thought helpful?

- What evidence is there to support the thought?

- What evidence is there to disprove this thought?

Break down the information, gather evidence on the validity of each thought and align these thoughts with true ones. This allows us to dismantle the insecure beliefs that are so incredibly damaging. Thoughts can be deceiving. There is a delicate dance between soothing an overactive nervous system, bringing ourselves back to calm, and processing these complex situations surrounding our thoughts and feelings.

By changing our thinking, our experience changes.

When we think about uncertainties and unknowns, we feel the tension and fear attached. When we think about the possibilities of what may unfold, we feel the hope and excitement of the potential outcomes.

During this time, I often allowed the uncertainty fueled by my anxiety about the unknown and lack of control to get the best of me. Recalibrating our thoughts throughout this experience enables us to move forward with perspective and awareness of the impact of these thoughts and our capacity to influence them. Let's dismantle some lies.

THE LIES

LIE #1: MY PLAN IS THE BEST PLAN

―――∽∾∽―――

"When life gets blurry, adjust your focus" – Unknown

Hindsight has a way of bringing life into perspective in a way that living in real time can't.

If I knew then what I know now, my experience of infertility would have been much smoother. Perhaps a similar experience comes to mind for you, one in which things would be so different if you only had the insight that lived experience can give you.

That's what life is all about – learning and growing as we navigate through the complexities of it all.

During our fertility treatments, I was so caught up in the process of it and working towards the end goal of getting pregnant that I was losing sight of the bigger picture. Our goal was to build a family.

Perspective is a function of experience.

If I knew then, back at the start of my infertility journey, we would pursue an international adoption with such excitement and anticipation, what a different experience it would have been! If only I had known that the pain and suffering we were experiencing along the way were stepping stones to strengthen our emotional health and mature our relationship. I would have seen that this was setting us up for building our family in this unique way. What a softer experience it would have been. If I had known these things then, I would have loosened my grip on how things should play out for us; there would have been a softening of the rigid expectations seemingly set in stone. There would have been an openness to how things were *meant* to play out for us. Yet we learn from these challenges.

We simply cannot see it all when we're in the middle of it. We don't hold the broader life perspective and design, no matter how much we falsely believe we do or not. The reality is that many things in this world are out of our realm of influence or control. Whether you believe in God or another higher power, there are some things you cannot control. There is a comfort in accepting that some things are not within your power to change. For me, my faith helped me to accept this truth. There's an illustration on perspective where you hold a large photograph up to your nose, forcing your eyes to zero in on the small section of the photo in immediate focus. That small piece of the picture is in focus and can be seen clearly. With an emphasis on a small portion of the image, the bigger picture remains blurry and not in our awareness. As you move the photo further away from your face, your ability to see that small image in the context of the much broader view improves.

What was once blurry and out of focus is seen clearly, allowing the initial narrow view to be seen in the context of its more expansive landscape. It creates understanding. This phenomenon was experienced along my journey.

When current circumstances are viewed in the greater picture, we gain valuable insight that helps to loosen our grip on what we can't control. The "unknown" aspect of infertility is one of the most significant barriers to accessing a perspective outside our current circumstances.

We can't see what we don't know.

The swirling thoughts and feelings stemming from a limited *perspective* can be challenging to navigate, as it's built on little *knowledge*. It's brutal that we simply can't know this critical information. Questions like:

- Will I ever be out of this infertility vortex? If so, how long will this insanity last?

- If this treatment doesn't work, what will I do?

- If I have to do IVF, will I be able to cope?

- How will I feel or respond if (insert person's name) gets pregnant before me?

- Will I be able to manage the financial burden?

- Can I handle what's ahead?

- What will happen if I never become a parent?

- How will my relationship handle this strain?

When we cannot access answers to questions that can't be known when we desperately want answers, it stirs up so much discomfort.

I've learned that feeling comfortable with *being* uncomfortable is like a muscle that needs to be exercised regularly to manage the burden of the unknown.

No matter how I analyzed it, I could not have the whole story, and it could only unfold in time. Not in my time or my schedule, but in its own time. It's impossible to know how things will play out, no matter how much time is spent analyzing the situation.

Trusting that the bigger picture was known beyond myself brought me a sense of peace, even just a glimmer in times of despair. I didn't know how this hurt would be used for good, but I found a sense of peace in trusting there was a greater purpose and plan for it all.

This concept may play out differently for you. Regardless of your beliefs about how the universe works, it's helpful to acknowledge that we have a limited perspective, and there are limits to what we can control. There is freedom in surrendering to this lack of control, as we aren't meant to know it all.

Living childless began to feel like an undeserved punishment and a substantial delay in my life's plan. I would often get caught up in a destructive thought storm of "Why me?" as I watched others build and complete their families, still uncertain if I would ever be so fortunate. A thought process shift that I developed over time was to view the efforts we were exerting as working along the trajectory of growing our family. We didn't have a clear direction or a known destination, but our movement was an effort in the forward direction as our story was unfolding.

My husband would regularly caution me from putting my emotions and energy into the current treatment round that we were in and instead remember that we were working towards having a family as our ultimate goal. We would remind ourselves that within five(ish) years, we will have a child, however that came to be.

We were in the process of building our family, moving forward, learning as we went, and as treatments came and went. We were living life in real-time with the hope of what was to come. While a specific timeline or outcome wasn't a guarantee, it was an acknowledgment that we were moving on a path towards our goal, which is genuinely what mattered most. That was what we could control at the time: our broader focus on a family, not the immediate outcome. His words were likely motivated to ease the discomfort and calm my stress levels and the intense pressure I was placing on my body to resolve an unknown "issue." However, it was true and something I needed to be reminded of regularly. They were important words to hear, and some lessons take time to percolate and settle in.

When we view things differently, our experience of our situation changes. Viewing life from a positive lens is my natural wiring; however, the experience of infertility caused me to become easily discouraged in an uncomfortable way. With purposeful intention,

I began shifting my mindset towards the greater purpose of our actions rather than basing my mood on the current set of circumstances we were in. Viewing this stage of life through a broader perspective was wildly helpful in understanding deeper meaning, easing the emotional turmoil, and enhancing my capacity to get through and sustain myself in these demanding times.

It was too easy to wallow in the circumstances of not yet arriving at a goal while perpetually discontented about never reaching the mark. This exact issue caused me to be a shell of who I once was for a time. It tarnished positive aspects of my life and prevented me from engaging in my life with the same zest I had before. It doesn't have to be this way. When we trust the greater picture and release the intense desire to control the journey, we make way for moving through this experience with some wiggle room to allow things to unfold in the way they are meant to.

There is hope in knowing that life can be viewed from a new lens, that there is a broader scope of your story that will become known *in time*. There is purpose in your pain; your story isn't over yet, and it might just be getting started.

Questions:

1. What have you had to grieve along the way towards building your family
2. How might seeing your current situation in a broader context change how you feel
3. Can you think of a challenge you've faced that has turned out to be helpful?

LIE #2: HAVING CHILDREN IS THE TICKET TO HAPPINESS

———— ⚮ ————

Most of our friends and family members have kids. When we started trying to conceive, very few of them did. It seemed like a cruel joke watching everyone effortlessly build their families while we were left in the dust to battle and wait for ours. The same week we began our fertility treatments, my two older sisters announced their pregnancies within two days (very delicately and respectfully, mind you).

It was a tough time, and it was hard to balance the conflicting emotions of being happy for my family while simultaneously feeling so sad for myself.

As time went on and treatments continued, we welcomed several babies from our close circle of friends and family. The initial news would always hit hard, sometimes excruciatingly so, and then we would fall in love with each of these little people once they arrived.

Have you felt that? That tug and pull of wanting to be happy for someone else but then also pained to the point of hurting on your own behalf? This was my first encounter with these intense conflicting emotions. It makes sense from the outside looking in, yet challenging to navigate through. At times I couldn't. I'd need to collect myself or remove myself from the situation to keep my feelings contained. It didn't feel okay at the time as it was so far from who I knew myself to be, yet looking back now, I wish I had given myself more grace in this area. We can all use a bit more grace in times of struggle.

As a result of being around so many little ones, we got a close and personal view of life with babies and young children. Life with a new baby seems to be a time of experiencing the most significant gap between expectation and reality. Babies are adorable and beautiful and exhausting and draining. What was mainly jealousy, frustration and sadness about ourselves slowly shifted to seeing the opportunity in our current situation. If pure happiness and fulfillment were on the other side of having a child, that would be one thing. But the truth is that life with a new baby is incredibly hard. It involves so much energy exertion, and emotional and physical drain all at once. It was clarifying and helpful for us to debunk these concepts of a misconstrued reality, the reality I was desperate for and felt I was missing out on.

Along the way, I equated having children with a perfect picture of happiness, and I thought being childless was a life sentence of loneliness and inadequacy. Children are not miracle workers, they don't solve all of life's issues, and they aren't magical beings of perfection. These very expectations mustn't be placed on them either – it's unfair and harmful to look at what we may gain over what we can give. They are exhausting, all-consuming, life-changing, and amazing all at once.

One summer evening, I was with a friend watching our husbands play baseball, and a meaningful conversation took place on the bleachers. I shared how inadequate and insecure I was feeling around my friends with children. The insecurity that stemmed from my childlessness brought up the feeling of falling behind in life as everyone around us was having children (like it's a collective race of some sort? What was I even racing towards?).

Motherhood can feel like an exclusive club for those of us struggling to join and hate being left out of. There is no "mama bear" shirt, no mom's groups, or entry into the "mamapreneur" markets. Being left out of a club that you're trying the hardest to get into is discouraging and hard.

My friend was legitimately surprised by how I felt and said, "Do you want to know what *we* are all thinking? We are jealous! We are jealous of the time you get to spend with your husband, your free time to yourself, the flexibility in your home life and the opportunities you have available."

Of course, no one was jealous that we couldn't conceive. Our friends and family with young children were in the throes of the authentic challenges of early parenthood. Their struggles were simply different, unique variations of demanding. We were energetic, and they were exhausted. We remained flexible while their schedules were rigid. We had free time when they didn't even have bathroom breaks alone.

When stuck in comparison mode, we must acknowledge the complete picture of what we are comparing against.

I needed to hear the other side. I needed the affirmation that everyone wasn't sitting around feeling sorry for me and looking down on me for not yet having children. I needed that outside perspective. And it was a great reminder to water the grass I was standing on and simply be where I was. Wherever we are in our lives, we won't know how long the current season will last or what the ending will look like. We can only change our response to our reality in real-time.

Seeing opportunity in a season of struggle is a game-changer. Having additional time in my waiting journey allowed me to take the time and opportunity to share my thoughts with you and process them for myself.

My goal soon shifted to making the best of my current reality while honoring the challenging parts along the way.

I had lived with this false idea that everything would feel complete and better with a child. In reality, there will be new challenges to face and new goals to work towards, and next steps that I will anticipate until the end of time. If we aren't careful, children can bring a new set of goals or milestones to chase: having your child sleep through the night, starting school, learning to drive, or even moving out.

There will always be something ahead to aim for and anticipate; it's human nature.

The phenomenon called *"hedonic adaptation"* is coined by psychologists Brickman and Campbell[2] to explain our tendency as human beings to chase happiness, only to return to our original emotional baseline after getting what we want. At one point in time, my current set of circumstances was precisely what I wanted – my house, spouse, and job. Our nature is to adapt to our new normals and chase the next "something" that offers just a little more happiness.

I am acutely aware of this in my own life. It can be an exhausting experience without awareness, and we risk missing out on the happiness right in front of us.

I can remember talking to my grandma about how I just needed to get through that next test, or that particularly stressful presentation, or that one big race, and then I'll feel good and be stress-free. We all know this is a moving target that is replaced with the next "thing" along the way, whatever that is.

In my grandmother's wisdom, she would remind me that it would ultimately just be something else that replaces my current set of obstacles or the "thing" I was striving for. She shared that I would have to work on settling into life in the here and now rather than chasing the next thing or finding relief in completing the next task.

Another concept by Harvard lecturer Tal Ben-Shahar defines the "*arrival fallacy*" as the "false belief that reaching a valued destination can sustain happiness."[3] He says that "attaining lasting happiness requires that we enjoy the journey on our way towards a destination we deem valuable. Happiness is not about making it to the peak of the mountain, nor is it about climbing aimlessly around the mountain; happiness is the experience of climbing towards the peak."[3]

So, while I don't know how long the climb will be, intentionally working on embracing the journey is the goal; the destination does not hold all the answers our mind can so easily lead us to believe we will find there.

At some point along the way, I realized that I didn't want to be sitting on my rocking chair at the end of my life, looking back at a young, healthy, vibrant time, knowing that I wished it away. "Fertile" years are vibrant years, some of the best of our lives. Time is our most precious, nonrenewable resource. There are no "do-overs" and no guarantees of how much time we will be blessed with.

I don't recall a specific moment during this season when I came to see this new perspective . However, I realized I had been allowing my circumstances to get the best of me for too long. It robbed me of my optimistic, naturally happy disposition and left me cynical and bitter. It required some serious reflection and a conscious switching of gears to appreciate the season we were in. Life is exhausting when you're perpetually dissatisfied. It was time to choose another type of "hard"; the kind of "hard" that helped me accept that this situation was difficult, and it was time to see the opportunities rather than waste them. I couldn't stay there any longer, and it was time to come to a place of acceptance and seek joy in the season I was in.

Arriving at a place of contentment was satisfying and relieving. Ridding myself of this imaginary list of obstacles blocking happiness was a helpful start. It was time to stop wishing for a fast-forward button during the challenges of life that would rob the joys that are right here in the present.

Erik and I opted to take advantage of our *bonus time* as a family of two by traveling, volunteering, connecting with friends, investing time into our families, and building relationships with our nieces and nephews. It has been such a unique and valuable time. Investing in ourselves and finding fulfillment in different areas of our lives allowed us to engage more fully in our lives. We were able to see this stage of life for what it was and all of the immense blessings created emotional freedom that I missed out on for a time while feeling stuck in the vortex of discontentment. Finding joy in the here and now is possible, even if it is so far from where you want to be. It meant taking the trip, joining the baseball team, signing up for the race, and seeking joy in day-to-day living.

I asked the online survey participants about what opportunities the experience of infertility offered them. There were common themes among the responses, which were so encouraging. In times of challenge, it can be helpful to look for opportunities.

Connection was a common theme among many responses. Connecting with others through the shared experience created friendships and meaningful support during a challenging time.

Personal growth and learning that some things in life are completely out of our control and the capacity to see life through a different lens.

Resiliency developed due to facing fears (needles), developing patience, and working through the challenges of infertility.

Empathy and compassion for self and others.

Career opportunities supporting others with the additional time without caring for a family at home.

A stronger relationship with a partner navigating the challenges of infertility together as a team.

Adoption and building a family in a different way.

Infertility can bring about opportunities when we are open to them.

Seeing current circumstances as an opportunity allowed me to see our life as it was in the moment, and it was pretty awesome. Life itself is such a gift, which is meant to be *lived*. There are no guarantees about it either. Our time could be up tomorrow. I'm not one to sit on the sidelines, and I don't think you want to be caught there either. I have been in a season of being childless and found joy and happiness. That *is* possible. The journey here was not easy, but it has been good: purposeful, meaningful, grueling, and really, really good.

You may have people in your life – a partner or extended family member – who believe that a child means happiness for you and them. I urge you to question what happiness means for you, just for you, and go from there. Having a child isn't the key to happiness. There is the possibility of finding steady ground while still waiting and living in the unknown of how your family may come to be. Be joyful in the hope of what is coming while exploring the opportunities available to you in *this* season.

A Message on Comparison

Comparison hinders our happiness. We know this to be accurate, yet it's so natural to fall into this mind trap. It takes a lot of self-awareness to redirect this patterned thinking when we find ourselves wrapped up in it. It's natural to compare ourselves to others, and there are times that it can be helpful to gauge how we are progressing.

Are we scoring at the top of the class or the bottom? The answers can give us essential information about focusing our attention while studying.

We live in a world that makes it too easy to be in constant comparison mode. It is easier than it's ever been to find out too much information about what someone else's life looks like without the well-rounded story of context to understand situations fully. It's easy to feel discouraged by the shiny look of others' highlight reels when we are intimately aware of our day-to-day challenges. We do this all the time.

Our thoughts are powerful, and the information we take in can promote helpful and positive thoughts or contribute to toxic thinking. They can influence and dictate our emotional health and how we feel. Learning the critical importance of intentionally taking captive all thoughts of comparison is vital to keeping our mental health in check. We must halt them in their tracks. These harmful thoughts of comparison can be treacherous during fertility treatments when stress is particularly heightened, hormones are being manipulated, and the stakes of current circumstances are so high.

Can you relate? It can be downright agonizing when you want something so much and see others around you living out your dream.

My triggers were pregnancy announcements, walking past pregnant women in public, seeing maternity photos on social media, pregnancy advertisements and commercials, and mainly being in the vicinity of conversations around family planning like it was all a simple choice.

Yup, there were a lot of triggers.

A spiral of negative thoughts would so quickly launch me into thought storms, "They've only been married for six months, and they're already expecting!", "They only had to endure two IUI cycles," "They aren't equipped financially to have another child," "They aren't as capable of a parent as I could be," and so on. Horrible thoughts led to awful feelings. Judgemental thoughts revealed more about how harmfully I was judging myself than how I was judging others. It was ugly. It feels ugly recounting these thoughts.

Hurting hearts have hurtful and harmful thoughts, and it requires mental gymnastics to manage the many triggers that prompt these cascades of thoughts and feelings. At the root of so many of these insecure feelings and judgments were my feelings of inadequacy and feeling "not enough." A mixture of jealousy, fear, pride, sadness, and grief would lead to harmful judgment and criticism of others and myself. It reminded me that I was "falling behind" with every pregnancy announcement like I was in a race.

Where that final race destination was, I am still not even sure.

I felt sure that I was not good enough and didn't measure up in the comparison game. It wasn't until releasing myself from the family planning comparison that I could dramatically turn my emotional experience around. It involved working diligently to catch myself in the act of comparison to release the thoughts. It sometimes required adjusting my social media feed to control some of the triggering information coming at me.

Social media is a highlight reel of people's lives.

We know that even for ourselves, we are posting about exciting, fun, upbeat, or funny things, and our emotions don't consider this reality when we are quickly scrolling through the content on our feed. The cute baby photos aren't always prefaced with the weeks of colic, no sleep, struggles with breastfeeding, or extreme mental fatigue surrounding them. The couple sharing pictures of their flashy vacation may be getting some reprieve from losing a loved one and needing to catch a breath.

The list of possibilities goes on.

We never know the whole story, which makes sense given the platform and its purpose of entertainment and connection. Research shows that the closer the degree of communication, calling someone on the phone or directly texting friends, is related to more positive outcomes than more distant connections like Facebook posts or Instagram stories that are more connected with negative feelings. These more distant connecting avenues are full of people's lives that we don't fully understand, which would otherwise allow us to see photos or videos in the greater context of their reality rather than as complete happiness and joy at *all* times.

When we know the fullness of someone's story, we can appreciate the cute baby photo as a glimpse of joy in their struggle or the vacation as a much-needed break for our friends. We don't naturally view all pictures in the context of their more in-depth story because we simply don't know it, and we are more apt to take things at face value.

When we put words to uncomfortable feelings, it helps release some of their power.

Talking about our feelings, as uncomfortable as they are to even admit at times, helps to dismantle them amid a mindset of comparison. Reminding ourselves that each person has their battle, their own story and no connection or influence on our own story can offer clarity and a safe degree of separation. It wasn't all about me. That glowing pregnant woman may be battling a disease, facing a financial crisis, grieving a loss in her life, or a woman who had silently been struggling with infertility. Or simply a happy pregnant woman is looking forward to expanding her family, which doesn't affect our family-building process, other than being painful to witness. Our stories are unique, and someone else's family building did not impact my own.

Comparison is never equal: it doesn't improve the situation in any way, it's based on many false assumptions, and it doesn't accomplish anything but foster the feeling of misery.

Viewing life from a place of scarcity and feeling like there is never enough makes it look like other people's lives are covered in glitter and our own lives sprinkled with dirt. When we shift our focus to observing others' experiences, we can have a more realistic view of our own experiences. Looking further outside of ourselves and current circumstances can help relieve the immediate tension in our lives. We can bring awareness to things going well that we can be grateful for, rather than only focusing on what we feel we lack.

When I came to the place of accepting that my life and journey would not be as I had expected, I was reminded that *no one's life is exactly as they expected it to be.* To be jealous of someone's fertility means that I must acknowledge the challenges in their lives. My life and my challenges are meant for me, they are part of what makes me, me, and another person's challenges are meant for them. We are all trying to exist and do the best we can in this crazy world.

Life is complex, and we are all trying our best to navigate it with the tools we have in our toolkit. There are no easy, straightforward comparisons, and what are we trying to accomplish by making these comparisons anyway?

Rather than using others as a measuring stick of our happiness, let's compare ourselves to who we were yesterday and work to be better with this in mind. Do we want to step on others' backs to feel okay? I certainly don't. It's a skewed measurement and is unhealthy, particularly in the realm of things we can't control.

Competition has been known to stimulate my motivation. It is my default setting in my personality, and I am working on ensuring I bring out its positives and release the negative aspects. It's not a good look. Ask anyone who has played recreational softball with me. In the fertility world, having a competitive nature has proven to be helpful – a fuel that kept my focus on the prize and enhanced the discipline required to follow through on rigorous treatment plans.

Combining competitive comparison towards other people and an outcome out of my control was a sour mix. I had made a recipe for defeat and a massive inferiority complex for myself.

Child-bearing years naturally surround us with pregnancy and babies. Infertility magnifies the awareness of pregnancy and children, just like buying a new car tends to increase the awareness and seemingly increases the number of similar vehicles seen on the road. What we focus on influences what comes into focus. Most of my extensive social and family network currently have or are expecting children, including many couples having conceived through IVF. If I didn't release the comparison, I would have continued to be emotionally uncontained. My time was spent feeling awful about my childlessness in a sea of children and feeling terrible about having these feelings. I've spent enough time there to know that it's not a fruitful way of living but rather a state of steady deterioration.

Someone else's fertility has nothing to do with anyone else's family, nor does their choice to have or not to have children or their ability and speed at which they can conceive. This shift came first out of necessity and then understanding its validity with experience. When you're trying so hard for something, it's natural to feel sadness, jealousy, anger, and frustration when you aren't getting what you want. It can be near impossible to separate your personal emotional experience from others' joy and celebration.

We can learn from each other's experiences and think through another's experience and how it might feel to be in their shoes, but comparing and competing frankly isn't helpful. Judging others isn't helpful either. Full stop. When I compete with those around me, I aim to catch myself, speak kind words to offer compassion in challenging times, and redirect these thoughts. Being honest about struggles makes someone a more relatable human being. We all have struggles; some are more visible than others, but none of these struggles negate our worth.

We all have a story, insecurities, and areas we feel we don't quite measure up. This means we are human. Spending all of our time fixated on our own experience holds us back from being our unique selves, impacting our ability to connect with others. Focus on the connection over comparison. Connect with others, but don't see them as a measuring stick.

Questions:

1. Ask yourself, how do I feel about my current state of childlessness?
2. What opportunities does my current family dynamic offer?
3. What are five things that I am grateful for?
4. What can I do to move even a percentage closer to how I want to feel in this season of waiting?
5. What are your comparison triggers?
6. For the next 30-days, start the day off by writing down three things you value about yourself.
7. When you catch yourself comparing, stop and

acknowledge your thoughts and feelings, then challenge yourself to see the whole picture. Are these thoughts true? Are they helpful? What's a more balanced thought process in light of the facts rather than the feelings behind it? Consider documenting these thoughts and feelings and challenging them.

LIE #3: THE FUTURE IS OURS TO CONTROL

In the days of self-actualization, motivational speaking, and seizing the opportunities in life, I believed that I had total control of my life. The harsh reality of infertility was coming to learn that this was not true. I could, however, control how I went through the process, my mindset, and being open to other possibilities, but I couldn't control the exact outcome, no matter how hard I tried.

As discussed earlier, we worked towards seeing the opportunities while going through our season of waiting. Travelling became something we enjoyed with our extra time. One year my husband and I went on a winter vacation to Morocco to experience a different culture and part of the world – a trip that was much easier with just the two of us. It was full of adventure and a jam-packed schedule to see all the sights. We had a great time, ate fantastic food, and enjoyed a highlight moment of riding camels in the Sahara Desert, where we camped out for two nights.

Our connecting flight home was grounded for a night. The

airline provided us with vouchers for taxi rides to a hotel and vouchers for dinner and breakfast to cover the additional meals of the trip. Looking back, the process was truthfully seamless. The difficulty came from the fact that we didn't know what was happening from the initial delay to when it was sorted, about five to six hours later. We waited four of those hours under the impression that our flight was simply delayed. At that time, the changing information slowly trickled in, ultimately announcing the cancellation of our flight.

The fascinating part of this experience was observing how people around us reacted throughout the "in-between" time, oscillating between complete confidence that we would be making it home that night and the likelihood of staying the night at a hotel on a small island off the coast of Portugal. Before receiving any news from the airline during our delay, there were whispers from people, making up stories to fill in the gaps of missing information. One gentleman was concerned we would be stranded on the island for a week, hearing a rumor that flights to Toronto only took off once a week from the island we were on. Another theorized that the pilot was intoxicated and unfit to operate the plane. Again, not one piece of factual data had been shared.

Erik and I discussed early on during the delay that we couldn't control the outcome of the flight, so we would just kick back and see how it all played out, dealing with any consequences or happenings as they came up with available information; no theories or hearsay. We were some of the more relaxed people at the gate. We'd had much experience with waiting things out that we couldn't control at this point. I have not always been so smooth and calm in the midst of uncertainty.

In the online survey, I asked what one of the most significant challenges of infertility had been. One woman stated, "The realization that no matter how hard you work at it, how much of yourself you pour into the process, what you change and modify in your life to make it possible, and how badly you want it, or how many times you try, there are many elements that are out of your control, and there is no guarantee." The unknown is incredibly scary, and we are desperate for certainty in times that it doesn't exist.

Altogether, I've spent too much time collectively strategizing and guessing what may happen with the information I could not know. I would strategize during a treatment cycle as if the cycle had already failed. I would plan to ease the potential disappointment and soothe the desire to know the next plan. This seemed to be the natural process, to anticipate and predict the outcome and never be a millisecond without a plan in place. The reality? We can't know what we don't know. Statistics can give us an idea of what things *might* be like for the population, but they do not tell us precisely what we will experience. There is no data more relevant than the data point we live and add to that data set. Some things can seem so sure and ultimately fail. Other things can rally against all odds and come out victorious. I've seen these scenarios play out with friends going through infertility.

While the strategy of anticipating failure helped to pacify the anxiety of the unknown at that moment, it didn't change the disappointment. It didn't erase the uncertainty or smooth over the pain. It certainly didn't change the outcome. Those emotions still had to be felt and processed. I tried to escape my feelings during treatment cycles by being armed with information, a plan, and a clear strategy.

For me, thinking is more manageable than feeling. It was more of an emotional distraction, a way to avoid the discomfort of the uncertainty and replace it with logical thinking. Anticipating an uncertain outcome does not ease the pain. There is a common misconception that the results of a probability experiment will affect the results of subsequent trials. If we flip a coin and get heads the first time, people often think this means that tails will be more likely if you flip a coin a second time, which is not true. Each time you flip a coin, the chance of getting heads is 50%, and the possibility of getting tails is 50%. The previous results don't impact the probability of getting an outcome on any given trial.

There is this misconception that we can play with statistical data. The data set tells us what has happened for a group of "data points" in the past, and we can extrapolate what is "likely" to occur from the data set, but it doesn't impact the chances for a given individual data point. Fertility treatments result in binary outcomes, a positive pregnancy test or not. It will either work or it won't. I spent a lot of time playing around with the statistical data in my mind and wasted a tremendous amount of energy doing it.

When information is missing, we fill in these gaps with our best guesses – it's naturally what our brain does. Trying to clarify uncertainties helps provide a sense of control over what feels like disorder or chaos. Information filters best in our brain when its flow is smooth, complete, and tied off in a bow.

Knowledge helps us feel grounded and prepared with a plan. Not knowing an outcome leaves us feeling uncertain and uncomfortable with gaps in information and a sense of being in limbo. There is general unease.

The tighter the passengers at the airport clung to getting on a flight and home that night, the more challenging the flight delay and cancellation was to accept. The highly-stressed passenger had to wait in the same airport, in the same lines, and stay at the same hotel an extra night like everyone else. Clinging tighter to the desired "plan" didn't magically change the flight, and it only made the process of waiting more miserable.

For years, I had to work to find joy in my life that wasn't going my way. Feeling sorry for myself didn't change the outcome, and wanting it more than the people next to me didn't change the result. Outcomes we can't control will play out as they are meant to. We can control how we process and accept deviations and pivoting plans. Taking some control over our experiences in how we process them before the experience takes us over is the name of the game.

Rigid expectations are not an infertile woman's friend. The tighter we cling to the outcome, the more resistant we become to changing course. Finding that balance between rigidity and chaos is the sweet spot. Flexibility and open-mindedness allowed our changing story to unfold more freely. Most paths in life are not linear, and straight lines are dull, anyway. Unpredictable and zigzagging paths are the most adventurous. Take ownership over your adventure.

Questions:

1. What is one thing that I can work on to stop planning/controlling?
2. What would it look like to be more flexible during this season of waiting?
3. Ask yourself, what experiences or opportunities would I like to explore? Connected to fertility or not.
4. What is one small thing that you can let go of while waiting?

LIE #4: INFERTILITY IS A SEASON OF BEING STUCK

When life is smooth sailing, it can feel pretty great, right? When you move through an amusement park on a low-traffic day or travel home from work and hit every green light, gosh, that feels good. Choppy waters are unsettling – they require strategizing and alertness. Calling in extra support when your computer starts acting up or navigating an injury that slows your momentum creates disruption. Being stuck, unable to move forward, is hard. In March 2020, when the pandemic struck, I went from seeing patients in my office one day to not being able to go to the office the next. Momentum came to a complete halt. It's disorienting and overwhelming at the same time. The comfort of progress and staying in the natural rhythm of life were halted entirely. It takes time for the mind to catch up with it all. We will all remember this time in our lives and its impact at that time.

Some seasons in life can feel smooth – that sense of fulfillment and forward motion, when we feel vibrant and vital. Other seasons are choppy or downright leave us feeling stuck; they are murky and muddled, confusing and complicated. Infertility was a time that caused me to feel completely stuck in a way I had never experienced before. The human experience involves a variety of seasons, although I wasn't prepared for how jolting it was when my forward motion came to a dramatic halt.

Feeling stuck was an unusual predicament. I was deep in the mud, still breathing air, but with capacity for little else. It wasn't a good look any more than a good feeling. I was stuck in the reality that I had to follow specific protocols, and stuck in the rigidity of appointment times and treatment dates. I was stuck understanding that this was my life and not some alternate universe. This couldn't be my life. There were times when I would say to myself, "This can't seriously be happening to *me*," even years into the process. I felt like a victim of my circumstances. Everything halted and circled around infertility.

This feeling was hard to shake. The process of fertility treatments takes up so much time and energy. There isn't much wiggle room between the strict timing and scheduling of ovulation testing, medication timing, treatment schedules, early morning clinic trips for bloodwork and ultrasounds in IUI or IVF procedures. Hours later, I would find out the medication protocol, and I sometimes required injections within hours of a phone call. I couldn't live longer than hours in that season without physically completing the necessary protocols. The situation forces infertility to constantly be top-of-mind, like a leash reining in any thoughts of freedom. I remember driving my sister-in-law and her friends for her bachelorette festivities one evening. That 10 p.m. cell phone buzzer rang, and I had to "tactfully" pull the car over, sharing that I needed to give myself medication (preparing and administering a needle). There were no private bathrooms to hide away in this scenario. It didn't fit the tone of the evening to share the purpose of my actions. I just completed the task, had feelings of shame and embarrassment, and moved on. Fortunately, the ladies picked up the tone and allowed me the space to do what I needed to do, and we went on with the fun evening. As usual, I wanted to live my life, social engagements and all, but the reminders pop up and invade these sacred spaces of life as I knew it.

In talking to a close friend about this concept of feeling stuck, she likened her experience to being in a mountain bike race, and you're the only one who got caught in a giant mud hole, unable to get out. You just have to struggle with your bike, watching others race past you. It's defeating, disheartening, and feels unfair. It knocks the wind right out of you, but you keep going. You keep struggling because, without the struggle at that moment, you just stay exactly where you are, and yet the race is still on.

The stuck feeling intruded on both my inner dialogue and my social calendar. It can be a pervasive, parasitic experience if we aren't careful. For a while, it felt like it was controlling my life. The "What if I'm pregnant?" question was the filter used for making so many decisions. "Should I get a snowboarding pass this winter? Better not, I might get pregnant", "Should we play baseball this summer? Let's think about it, it may not be a good idea if pregnant", "Should I train for this race? It might be too hard on the body during treatments". These thoughts amplify the intense feelings of failure with each passing month as it gets mixed with the disappointment of missed opportunities. The goal of pregnancy was not fulfilled, but it came along with the reality of missing out on a season of fun snowboarding or whatever activity was passed up. Maybe you're missing out on some great things in your life too. Playing the "What if" game with every decision you make. It's disappointing and upsetting, isn't it? It's frustrating, confusing, and overanalyzing it all is exhausting.

It got tiring viewing life from this lens, especially when I never wanted to order these glasses in the first place. Critically analyzing everything through this unknown potential scenario that is so desperately wanted can be such a downer. Without much work, intense resentment can certainly build, and this building of bitterness was a caveat for me in making a change.

Decisions about spending free time, in addition to the already limited infertility lifestyle, led to resentment towards my situation and my own body. Something had to give. My decision-making process shifted from pausing to living, understanding that if and when a pregnancy took place, I would happily cancel plans, cancel that trip, or find a replacement for the baseball team. I remember consciously thinking that I couldn't keep living in these "what if" scenarios. Rather than seeing life as "what ifs," I would see life as it currently was and modify it if the situation changed. I felt tired of being stuck in this victim mindset and feeling sorry for myself. I couldn't trap myself anymore with this way of thinking. I don't remember when or even how this all shifted. It came down to choosing a different type of "hard." It was hard to view life through the "what if" and "poor me" lens, and it was hard to see the reality of the situation and move forward. Both were hard – I chose a "hard" that would better fuel my day-to-day living. Harboring resentment towards life was not a comfortable place to be. This mindset helped me minimize my regrets, and I wish the same for you.

Resentment would continue to build had I carried on the way I was and not engage in the activities that brought me joy. By saying "yes" to playing baseball in the summer, I could engage in a fun activity outdoors with friends, and it ended up being a terrific stress-relieving activity.

You can feel stuck in that you are not moving along as you originally planned or envisioned moving through this race. However, I have come to view the analogy of the race itself as problematic because life is not about getting from start to finish. The journey itself is most important, and our destinations can easily change. Infertility is not a pause. I was never stuck. There is a building of potential energy and hope waiting on the other end of this struggle. When an investment of our resources doesn't amount to a desired external result, we must take inventory of what potential is happening on the inside. This potential might very well be getting ready to launch into motion. No challenge we face or perceived pause in our plans is ever wasted.

When reflecting on that time now, it's hard to believe everything that this experience embodied. The amount of strength and grit that it takes to follow detailed plans and balance a constant yet inconsistently interrupted schedule while maintaining the routine of life is, quite honestly, remarkable. It is beyond challenging to carry on and fulfill responsibilities as though there isn't sustained grief, heartbreak, and reproductive trauma all going on simultaneously. It takes courage and resilience to travel this road. As I work with women facing infertility in a clinical setting, I often remind them of their strengths. It's easier to observe and reflect this from the outside looking in. It is incredible and powerful to witness the grit and capacity of a fighting, hopeful mother-to-be. I have so much more empathy and self-compassion when I reflect on my own experience than when I was in the throes of it all. We can't fully comprehend the complexities of our situations while in the midst of them. Feeling extremely tired and emotionally weak from the experience doesn't lend itself to the reality of the incredible strength it takes to carry on, injection after injection, day after day.

Do you know that stuck feeling? Let's think of it as the momentum building during the struggle before being propelled forward into something extraordinary. The discomfort that exists while on the precipice of transformation. It's not a struggle; it's a shake-down. Shedding the unnecessary, reclaiming what is essential, and developing a renewed purpose for the pain. It turns out the very source of the stuck was the source of my hope. This strong desire to have a family on my timeline that kept coming up empty kept this hope alive. The hope of a family fueled the mission and allowed me to keep showing up. There was confusion in this dichotomy, and there was an unraveling in this kind of "stuck."

As the building momentum in the realm of fertility occurs, looking to other areas of life where growth is happening can be more immediately satisfying. As humans, we intrinsically desire growth and forward movement. Infertility can feel like stunted growth and enhance this feeling of falling behind. We can have a bit more control in other areas of life to offset this feeling of being stuck in a straightjacket of circumstances. Some considerations may be working on a new skill, reading a new book, or volunteering in your community. It may even mean something as significant as a career change or starting a new education program for some. Having a different focus working on something with a more linear path can help soften the challenge of accepting this momentum-building time. There can still be a slight twinge in my gut when I feel like the pace of my life isn't lining up with what I had planned or when I feel like others around me are progressing faster. It takes regrouping and reminding myself to shed the comparison game and stay in my lane. Our lives are unique to us as individuals. We aren't meant to live anyone's life except our own. Life happens on our own timeline, with our own lessons learned, and on our path to who we are meant to be. The pace and process are exactly as they should be.

Let's give ourselves permission to lean into the pause to regroup and reorient ourselves in the face of feeling stuck. If we get right down to it, our days on this earth are numbered, and we don't know what tomorrow holds. This knowledge should enhance the urgency that we need to live today. Life is full of twists and turns with absolutely no guarantees.

My stepmom had a sudden, massive brain aneurysm during our treatments and spent 18 days in a coma without much hope of survival from her medical professional team.

Miraculously, she survived and is a well-loved part of our family, affectionately "Gigi" to our team of littles in the family. All that mattered was spending quality time with loved ones at that time. Life was very quickly and abruptly put into perspective. We don't know what we will face, which is more reason to remind ourselves of what we have right now. That we need to live right now. Recounting all that we are grateful for and blessed with and not fixating on where we want to be is critically important in pursuing joy and happiness in this hard season.

Questions:

1. What areas of your life are you feeling stuck in?
2. Are there feelings of resentment building in certain areas of your life?
3. If you can "unpause" one crucial area of your life for your sense of well-being, what would it be?
4. What is one way you have seen forward movement during this season?
5. What have you learned about yourself that you're proud of?"

LIE #5: INFERTILITY IS A LONE JOURNEY

With infertility being as common as it is, one would expect it to feel more commonplace and less lonely than it actually feels. It felt incredibly lonely in the early stages until I learned the critical importance of being in a supportive community. Shame kept me from being open and honest about my infertility with others, and I found myself disconnecting from people around me.

Spending time with others became filled with emotional triggers that felt overwhelming at times, interfering with my ability to enjoy myself and, at times, my ability to feel okay. I was caught up in the negative inner dialogue of my own experience that enhanced this invisible barrier I felt between myself and others. This perpetuates isolation and loneliness. These challenges started impacting my social life as my capacity to engage with others in the midst of building their families diminished.

Disconnection leads to loneliness and isolation; we are designed for connection and community. Loneliness, heightened emotions, physical discomfort, and fertility medication side effects combined can very easily lead to feelings of despair. Have you felt that? You're not alone. When you put all the pieces together, it can bring context to these feelings. These feelings are valid, and these feelings are complicated.

While in treatments, I'm sad that I went months without talking to some close friends after they became pregnant. It's pretty clarifying in hindsight just how emotionally taxing this was for an otherwise highly-social and engaged friend. The lack of connection was a barometer for my well-being at the time. It felt nearly impossible to keep my personal experiences and emotions separate from the joy I felt for my cherished friends and family while building their own families. I couldn't separate them and hadn't learned the validity of holding space for two conflicting emotions.

It felt natural and easier to simplify and close in my social network. It felt too painful, and I lacked the self-awareness to have meaningful interactions with those in a different stage of their family building. Emotional burnout is real, and these were protective mechanisms I had in place to function. I can see that now. I needed to close in to conserve energy, as there were no reserves left to expend the very little energy I had to manage the enhanced social drain.

Hindsight highlights the depth of a journey. My capacity for holding space for others' pregnancy joy had bottomed out. This was a season of turning down baby shower invites, hangouts with friends and family at times, and phone calls left unanswered if I didn't have the energy. At the time, I was in emotional preservation mode. My cup was empty, and I had nothing left to pour. In extreme overwhelm and distress, my energy resources were needed inward to get through the day and the current tasks.

Looking back on this season with fresh eyes, the source of my loneliness was coming from a place of hiding my shame. I didn't feel I could connect with others in the ways I had before, and I felt like I was falling behind and on a completely different level.

I remember hosting a baby shower for a friend. That feeling of being alone was hard at the time, but hosting this shower was something I felt was essential to honor a friend. I structured the event more like a "girls spa night" rather than a baby shower to opt for a more relaxed feel, less structured than some showers can be. There was a moment when the conversation shifted to family building.

I remember people talking through their process of *deciding* how many children they had initially planned for and what they were currently thinking would be best for them. Instantly my breathing quickened, my stomach tightened, and I had the urge to run out of my own house. I felt alone in this room full of women. I felt singled out, even though no one talked to me directly. I felt embarrassed that these women could so freely engage in a conversation that felt light to everyone but had been weighing me down for years. Feeling so alone in moments like these highlighted my need for connection.

In feeling isolated in my circumstances, I needed connection from those who truly understood them.

At this time, I found myself gravitating towards and connecting with others sharing this infertility experience. Connecting with people through shared experiences helped normalize the complexity of the struggle involved with infertility. Speaking with women while waiting for appointments and exchanging numbers and texts to stay informed on how treatments were going were constructive ways to feel supported and offer support.

These connections validated the emotional turmoil, as they would often express very similar feelings to me about various challenges. It can feel awful to experience grief after someone shares their exciting pregnancy news, and it can be hard to turn down a baby shower invite to a close friend because you can't sift through the complex emotions of it all. It's more accessible when you have someone to normalize these feelings with. Dr. Jannel Phillips, a neuropsychologist, says in the article, How Coping with Grief Can Affect Your Brain: "several regions of the brain play a role in emotion, including areas within the limbic system and prefrontal cortex. These involve emotional regulation, memory, multi-tasking, organization and learning. When you're grieving, a flood of neurochemicals and hormones dance around in your head. There can be a disruption in hormones that results in specific symptoms, such as disturbed sleep, loss of appetite, fatigue and anxiety."[4]

One of the recommendations Dr. Phillips[4] makes for grief is getting support through shared experiences, which often leads to sharing resources and strategies to help manage life during these tough times.

Our brains crave this level of connection during times of grief and distress. Shared experiences are the antidote to loneliness. Fertility clinics are bursting at the seams with couples facing infertility. Walking into a busy fertility clinic is a great visual representation that allows us to dismantle the inherent lie that we are alone in this battle. These people in the waiting rooms were living their life revolving around their menstrual cycle as well, other people's life plans and dreams were equally uncertain, and they were processing the complexities of it all at the same time I was. There is strength in numbers. While you'd never wish the experience on anyone, there is comfort in knowing you aren't alone. Being surrounded by other women experiencing infertility brought comfort and the sense of community I needed at this time in my life.

A group of women from our fertility clinic started a Facebook group to connect with women in the community to keep up-to-date on how everyone was doing between appointments. I kept in contact with two women in particular; we enjoyed dinners out together from time to time, processing our experiences and sharing with one another. There is camaraderie when you surround yourself with people who understand your struggle. Being heard and fully understood is such a gift. Are you having a tough day? Share with someone who understands it or will try their best to understand. I think this act of sharing helps lighten the load, both for the person sharing and for the person listening who might have been feeling something similar. Feeling overwhelmed by the medication and appointment schedule? Speaking with others who get it can neutralize the stress. Someone saying "I hear you," or "I felt that exact same way last week," or "I'm so tired of this too" validates the feelings that arise, allowing the frustration to come and go. Connection and being understood can allow the most uncomfortable emotions to be normalized. Rather than camping out with these emotions, we can simply ride the wave and let it pass. Even though we can feel alone, we are never alone. Infertility can feel lonely. It's crucial to find ways to reach out and connect with others to pacify this.

Social connection and engagement may change along this journey. Among the many voices in our heads, one to be particularly aware of is the "should" voice. Those voices tell us how we should feel or what we should do. I should have gone to the baby showers. I should have spent time with my friends and family during their pregnancies. I should have been more enthusiastic with pregnancy announcements. I've learned that "should-ing" can be used to remind us of the need for self-compassion in those moments. In reality, if I could have effectively been an active participant in a baby shower, I would have been there. At that time, I couldn't, and that's okay. It's also okay if you can celebrate with others. It's okay if you can't. What we feel is okay, even if it's not how we want to feel. When circumstances change, the ways we connect with others may change too.

I am so fortunate to have sisters to walk through life with. During this season, they supported the many ups and downs faced. They were there to listen to understand what I was going through. They were sensitive toward my situation as they were simultaneously building their families. They were a phone call away at all hours of the day while I was processing various pain points in real-time. They provide a richness to life and a sense of security. There were still times when connecting with them was hard. Looking back on this experience, I will forever be grateful and always know how deeply they love me because of how they handled this season in my life, with love, grace, and loads of compassion.

Even with this support network, I found it easy to feel alone. Understanding that others struggle with the same issue and feeling a sense of community around the issue are two different things. It takes work to build a community of people around this shared infertility experience that may not be comfortable or readily available to you where you are. Take some time to understand your needs and what resources or community groups are available in your area; these are helpful places to start.

There is an infertility support group in my town that I connected with. It's remarkable how much comfort is experienced when strangers discuss their unique versions of a shared experience. Shared challenges are a social equalizer. It is surprising the resistance that we often feel pushing ourselves to attend group meetings like this. I felt that way too. It's an "outing" of your struggle, which can feel awkward to do. When we walk into a space where everyone is facing their version of a battle, a unique offering of support exists in simply sharing space with one another.

Self-acceptance and owning my humanness were the key to connecting with others during this time. Acknowledging that to struggle with infertility was nothing to be ashamed about, any more than someone facing any other medical condition, like diabetes, cancer, or a broken bone. It involved accepting the fact that to struggle is to be human. Accepting ourselves and our needs each step of the journey helps open us up to others facing the same challenges. Self-compassion supports meaningful connection, and connection dispels loneliness.

Questions:

1. Do you find yourself pulling away from friendships? If so, how does that impact you?
2. What local infertility support groups or online forums are available to you?
3. How can you work to build connections while honoring your current capacity?
4. What are two small ways to reach out and connect to others you feel comfortable around? (e.g., chatting with someone while you wait for an appointment OR sharing with someone close to you that you are experiencing infertility)

LIE #6: INFERTILITY = INADEQUACY

Back in our early dating years, I had come home from university over Halloween weekend to visit my now husband, Erik. That night, we met up with some friends to go out for a dress-up Halloween dinner. We took an ironic approach to our costumes and dressed up as an elderly couple. We felt silly, fun, and proud of our detailed matching Halloween attire. That was, right up until we joined our friends at the restaurant. Let's just say they took the "attractive" Halloween costume approach, and we stood out a little more than we planned on. It's funny to look back on, as most embarrassing moments are, but it felt uncomfortable and awkward at the time.

Have you ever felt blatant inadequacy or not quite meeting the mark? It doesn't feel good, does it? It took quite a while before realizing that inadequacy was taking over my thoughts during this season of my life. Being in a room with everyone and their kids would have me crawling on the inside from simply feeling like I wasn't good enough because I wasn't at that stage of life. I didn't fit into some of the conversations either, which exacerbated these feelings.

I did not measure up to a bar that I had set for myself.

The sheer volume of tangled emotions makes it difficult to differentiate and tease out feelings and their origin. Everything feels terrible, and participation in these feelings is forced; no one signs up for it. I felt like my body wasn't working as it should, and I felt broken. This simply is not true. Being infertile does not disqualify you in any way or mean you aren't good enough. The experience of infertility lends itself too easily to making this feel true. The litany of tests, the consistent stream of "negative" or "failed" cycles, and the ever-changing medical protocols with the hope of manipulating an uncooperative body all amplify this. Even an otherwise confident person can quickly have their self-esteem and self-worth chipped away to believe that inadequacy is part of the story. This experience wore me down over the years and made me feel like *I* was a failure.

Untangling self-worth from fertility is critical. This was a crucial step in my healing and reacquainting myself and my worth as separate from my productivity or ability to become pregnant. We set our goal, made a plan, re-worked the plan several times along the way, and yet never felt any further ahead from where we started. When you bang your head against a brick wall enough times, it starts to throb. Not being able to move forward from this experience of infertility was tiring. I felt like I didn't measure up each time I came up empty. Others around me were having children, which stirred up jealousy and discontent within me. It felt awful, like wearing a heavy, wet blanket while it appears everyone else is prancing around in sundresses in the summer. It clouded my mind and my interactions. It caused me to feel insecure and inadequate.

Infertility does not impact the value of a human being. Being human is the prerequisite for intrinsic value, purpose, and worth. Fertility status does not define worth. I am human; therefore, I am valuable. You are human; therefore, you are valuable. Fertility does not dictate value, which is a fundamental concept so easily skewed during this time.

I have met so many amazing women at various clinics through my journey and professionally in my office. Never once have I looked down on these women for not getting pregnant. Not for even one second did I view them as inadequate or "less than" because of this struggle. If anything, I could see their incredible strength and courage as they fought month after month for the hope of growing a family. The level of resiliency demonstrated when things didn't work out, and their persistence as they kept trying is admirable. Reflecting on how I viewed others and becoming aware of my self-talk was an essential part of my process. Another plug for self-compassion. When we offer ourselves the same level of compassion that we do others, we can soften this experience monumentally:

- Extending the same grace and kindness, we offer to others can drastically change our own experience.

- Bringing awareness to our thoughts and self-talk.
- Bring understanding to where we are emotionally raw.
- Questioning whether or not we would speak to those we love in the same way we talk to ourselves brings context and helps us adjust our self-talk.

Learning to treat ourselves with the same kindness and compassion we treat others provides the space and grace needed to walk a challenging road.

As this awareness became clear that I wasn't judging other women facing infertility, it allowed me to release the judgment I was placing on myself and the perceived judgement I felt others were putting on me. We are told to treat others the way we want to be treated, and some of us need to treat ourselves the way we treat others, with kindness, compassion, and love. As women, we far too quickly put ourselves down when we need to be building ourselves and those around us up. We are valuable and worthy.

Speaking about our feelings of inadequacy can help dissipate them. Ugly thoughts that we harbor start to burrow in our minds and take hold, and these challenging thoughts become amplified in the dark.

After my husband and I finished our second and final round of IVF, we gave ourselves two months to regroup individually. We allowed ourselves to process our experience without the pressure of talking it through with one another. After this grace period ended, we had our first conversation about the next steps for us while out for a walk with our dog, Buddy. I hadn't planned on it, but I ended up sharing how I felt the burden of our infertility as it was likely a concern on my end. By simply sharing this with Erik, he reassured me that this process was one we entered into and are coming out of together. There was no blame, and there was no "you" and "me." It was us, and we were facing this season together. I released those harmful untrue feelings by expressing my feelings of inadequacy within our marriage. Sometimes we don't know the weight of these thoughts until they are gone.

Infertility can make you *feel* inadequate, but infertility doesn't dictate worth.

Questions:

1. Have you suffered from feelings of inadequacy?
2. What situations trigger these feelings for you?
3. What are three qualities your partner or best friend loves about you?
4. Activity: Create your own daily positive affirmation.

LIE #7: INFERTILITY IS
MY IDENTITY

———— ❧ ————

Our identity involves the many qualities that make us unique, those collected through experiences, history, and personality that make us who we are. A mosaic of puzzle pieces, with space for future pieces to fill in the gaps and add to the beauty of the ever-evolving picture. We consciously and subconsciously have thoughts about our identity, who we are, and the direction we aim to travel. When this is challenged, it can affect us at a core level.

Socially, women bear the weight of producing offspring, which can become intertwined with how we feel about our identity. We can never really determine the complexity of our deeply-rooted thoughts and expectations on this until we face an experience that challenges this identity. Not all women accept childbearing as part of their identity. However, many of us grapple with this unknown element of whether or not that piece of us will be actualized while undergoing fertility treatments. Among this group of women, some will become mothers through different avenues, and some never will, thus requiring a dismantling and rebuilding of our identity. Some of these thoughts and ideas are overt, and others are subconscious. I don't think I knowingly understood my identity to have any connection to childbearing until I was known to be infertile. This stirred up thoughts and challenges with my identity at that time.

The impact of infertility on my identity was significant. This unraveling process took time for me to figure out. Maybe it's impacting you too. I didn't understand all of this until I was on the other side of it all. Being in a group of women at a baby shower caused me to feel like a misfit. Playing baseball, I'd feel more comfortable around our male friends while the women discussed their postpartum physical discomfort running to first base. It's all mixed in. Small collections of experiences have an impact. Understanding this and breaking it down allowed me to separate the facts from the fallacy.

Playing "house" was a favorite childhood game for many children. It's the game where you reenact the day-to-day living routine, which in our home, was a mother-and-child dynamic of play. Growing up with three sisters allowed for regular house play. It makes sense: we model what we see, and what we experience makes an imprint on who we are and what we may wish to become. One of the most influential people in my life was my mother, so naturally, being a mother was something I thought about and anticipated with certainty of becoming. It is such a mixture of biological design and desire, personal expectation without a reason to challenge, and the underlying social expectation that all play a role.

Our ability to conceive does not define us.

It seems simple and obvious, and those outside of the situation likely can't make sense of this challenging part of the infertility experience. However, I felt less feminine, broken, and inadequate for these deficits, which felt uncomfortable. As an otherwise confident, competent woman, this knocked me down in a huge way – a way that was utterly unfamiliar and uncomfortable. Infertility interrupted the sense of security I felt regarding my own identity. Having children is not a prerequisite to being a woman or being a good person, and it is not a moral issue.

Socialization affects us even when we aren't aware of its intricate workings. When we face uncertainty and fear, it stirs up thoughts and emotions that cause us to understand ourselves and others in a whole new way. During my journey, I came across insecurity concerning my femininity. I did so without realizing how much our society, and myself personally, connected womanhood with motherhood as a mutually exclusive entity.

My memory doesn't include having experiences or conversations about gender or social expectations of men and women before our infertility struggle. It was never an area I'd given much thought to, how I related to being a woman. I never was made to feel less feminine because I loved athletics and competition during my younger "tomboy" days. These differences were celebrated in the same way that my sister enjoyed woodworking, singing, or operating farm machinery. As an adult, I am confident in myself and my unique intricacies, and I celebrate the people around me for their uniqueness. I can very readily remember feeling inferior and out of place during birth story conversations and feeling sick to my stomach when someone would say, "you're next!" regarding becoming pregnant in a lighthearted and fun way. Naturally, I felt less feminine without contributing and fulfilling this maternal role. Even now, I don't fully understand what that means and how I feel about it entirely. I just know that at the time, it caused me to feel even more insecure at a vulnerable time in my life.

It wasn't until my up close and personal infertility experience that I questioned these things concerning my female identity. To make matters worse, after several hormonal blood tests and evaluations, which typically came back unremarkable, I had one that was highlighted as abnormal. For a short time, I had elevated DHT (dihydrotestosterone) during my treatments, a form of testosterone. While it wasn't directly related to the challenges with fertility and didn't come with any symptoms, it made me feel incredibly insecure and shameful. Why did I have higher than normal levels of a primarily male hormone?

Speaking words to these things that would otherwise get stored up in secrecy and cause stress was the way I was able to work through it. I shared this with a few close friends and family members, and we made light of it and joked about it, which helped soften the experience. A couple of years after moving away from treatments, I was curious about my hormone levels and decided to get a health check. My DHT levels had completely normalized, offering the insight that it was likely a result of my treatment plan at that time. The interesting response was the relief I felt upon receiving these results. I didn't realize how much I was holding on to the awkward feeling of being even less feminine until I no longer had that story playing in the back of my mind. And really, even should those hormones have remained elevated, I know better than to let something as simplistic as a blood test define who I am. I hope the same for you. We are human beings, after all – complex and ever-changing human beings.

Connecting with other infertile women helped clarify and filter out some of these feelings. We are much more than our fertility status. Fertility is not the defining characteristic of femininity or our identity. Fertility is not a defining characteristic of worth, regardless of gender. I may always have a visceral response when in the throes of conversations about breastfeeding or birth experiences, as that won't be an experience I'll ever relate to or contribute to. We all have things that we can and cannot connect to based on our individual experiences. I can identify with others who have lost a parent but not someone experiencing chronic pain. I can identify with someone who has had a miscarriage, but not someone homeschooling four children. I can identify with someone who loves to run but not somebody passionate about drawing.

There are many ways in which we are different, but that doesn't make us inferior or superior to them. We are just different, with other likes and dislikes, different experiences, not different values as human beings. We each have our sensitive areas, and they are as unique as each of us is. When we know those areas of sensitivity, we can better prepare for and accept them as they come up.

I have learned that it's okay that I feel a pinch in my stomach during these sore spots in conversation when they come up. That doesn't make them bad or my reaction wrong; it's a piece of me and a reminder that I'm human, and it doesn't impact my identity. Knowing these areas for ourselves can help us rebound more efficiently by identifying our triggers and reminding ourselves of our truths while facing the moment's discomfort. When we listen to what makes our body react, we can move forward comfortably and offer ourselves compassion in the challenging moment.

It's okay to back away from these moments and know that you may need some recovery time afterward (we will discuss these situations and ways to establish boundaries later in the book). Honoring ourselves and our needs in times like this is an act of self-compassion.

Placing our identity in our circumstances is a path to adversity and discontentment. I've tasted life from there, and it isn't good. It's not fair to our emotional health to put so much pressure on outcomes we can't control, let alone have our identity wrapped up in it. When we take the experience of our hardships, lean into that discomfort of uncertainty, and allow ourselves to feel our way through it, we develop a deeper understanding of ourselves. Letting ourselves feel the hard feelings will enable us to process our experiences and integrate them into our life stories. It's an opportunity to strengthen our identities and learn what is true about us more concretely. These full experiences enhance our capacity as humans to care for and empathize with others.

When our identity is left to the changing and uncertain winds of infertility, it holds us back from being the people we were created to be. We can't hope, wish, or dream our way to a happily ever after that we long for so deeply. So, we are forced to dig deeper, to spend time seeing ourselves beyond the current set of circumstances.

Who are you meant to be *right now*? Not as a mother, not with the perfectly curated family you imagined, but *right now* in this process. Work on being that version of yourself. Don't let the unknown rob you of your joy and purpose in the present. Life as we know it is happening right now.

The season of reckoning and reconciliation after an identity crisis can result in the most brilliant resurgence of the person we are meant to become. In Brené Brown's[5] book, *Rising Strong,* she discusses a specific three-step process; First is the Reckoning: walking into our story; the second is the Rumble: owning our story; and the third, the Revolution: writing a new ending and changing how we engage with the world. When we've been shattered and broken, and our internal fire is dim, that's when the real magic happens. That's when we learn about what defines us and makes us unique. Not giving up, not giving in to the hopelessness of another failed cycle, not closing off to the world when you can't handle being around others, and moving forward at a different pace. That strength, sense of purpose, and burning desire to be better and make the world better are the defining pieces of the puzzle that make us whole. Not external circumstances, not the lack of response or heightened response of our physical bodies to various treatments, not the fear of the unknown. None of those is defining. The tenacity, grit, compassion, and empathy that this experience has elicited is where it counts. That's who you are. This is what enhances your confidence after spending the time dusting yourself off after the messy battle.

Infertility leads to many emotional states, not defining character traits; you are not your infertility. You, my friend, are so much more.

Questions:

1. What are three character traits that you like about yourself?
2. What do your friends and family love about you?
3. What is the most common positive feedback you get from others?
4. What is a trait you would like to work on developing? What are some practical steps to creating this trait?
5. What makes you, you? Develop a mind map of the things you value that make up your identity.
6. What is one thing that is fundamentally important to you/part of your identity?

LIE #8: NOTHING GOOD CAN COME FROM INFERTILITY

The Value of Self-Reflection

Life is relentless, and it passes us by quickly. It's our responsibility to capture the lessons that come our way as we journey along. The stress of infertility had me in an over-functioning mode. The pace of my life sped up as I raced from one task to the next. It was a season of a complete whirlwind, without wiggle room to reflect on how I was doing or knowing what I was even feeling most of the time. This was a coping strategy, a protective mechanism I put in place without being aware of it. There was no time to feel without stopping, which was a protective avoidance strategy. There is a tendency for many of us to busy ourselves in the face of stress and anxiety. I am good at packing a day full to the brim if I'm not paying attention. Avoidance is a tool to minimize the discomfort of feeling hard feelings. The downside to this was the limited time available to reflect on and identify what was needed.

It wasn't until treatments ended that I began to unravel the intensity of the experience and noticed some of the consequences of not taking care of myself during this time. I highly recommend that you give yourself permission to take the time you need to care for yourself during this period. Understandably, as the load in life is much heavier, you'll need more than you typically would to regroup.

Solitude is an intentional time of introspection and an opportunity to recharge, potentially providing valuable insight during this grueling season. This was a time that productivity as an avoidance tactic negatively impacted my ability to care for myself, resulting in exhaustion and burnout on the other end of it. Since this season has ended, I have learned the importance and life-giving power of solitude and self-care. A priest once told Brené Brown[6], "If you don't want to burn out, stop living like you're on fire." This struck a chord with me.

Life brings many challenges.

When challenging situations arise, making sense of or finding meaning and purpose in these challenges and times of suffering helps to bring purpose to it. Letting the tough stuff float by and moving on doesn't do the hardships justice, and it doesn't feel right. Before moving onwards in times like this, it can help to move inward. Drawing from experiences, learning from them, and finding meaning helps to bring purpose to our pain. It seems to sit better with me this way. We owe it to ourselves to grow stronger and wiser, rather than defeated and deflated from the obstacles we face in life.

For me, my faith in God offers support here. I draw on the hope of knowing that the challenges I face have purpose and play a role in the life planned for me. When we dig into purpose and meaning through times of suffering, it brings us hope for something more awesome yet to come and that no pain we experience on this earth is wasted.

The challenges throughout this experience have been responsible for the most significant growth. They have allowed me to learn a great deal about myself. Self-reflection is an essential component of development and has contributed to my capacity for gratitude towards my experience. There is so much to be thankful for. Personally, self-awareness brought a deeper level of self-compassion. When I became aware of the reality of what I was going through, what I needed, and how I responded to various stressors, I was able to show compassion to myself as I worked towards meeting these needs.

Self-awareness doesn't automatically help develop self-compassion, but it can bring understanding to oneself. Kristin Neff,[7] author of *Self-Compassion,* shares that self-compassion entails being warm and understanding toward ourselves when we suffer, fail or feel inadequate, rather than ignoring our pain or flagellating ourselves with self-criticism. Her book developed broader awareness on this important topic and was an excellent tool to learn and foster self-compassion.

Acknowledging how heavy some seasons are and their impact at that moment can create space and grace to tread through it gently. When we recognize that our capacity changes during challenges, we can adjust our expectations of ourselves in these times. Matching our capacity with our expectations can relieve a lot of frustration and personal turmoil that is felt when we can't perform in life in certain areas as we're bogged down by others. This understanding came well after the infertility offense; however, it has dramatically helped with the recovery period afterward. This has been a strong theme with my patients during the pandemic.

Self-reflection has been most rewarding for me during my darkest times, in the times where I've bent and nearly broken. It's been supportive in recoiling back to a more experienced self after those on-the-brink-of-breaking moments where I have built a more resilient and stronger version of myself. It's easy to stay stuck in the heaviness, yearning, and powerlessness of this experience, and I was there long enough.

Intentional living is critical. I had allowed self-pity, sadness, and despair to take hold. It took getting honest with myself in this situation and acknowledging that the current direction was not in alignment with who I wanted to be or who I was meant to be. Sometimes it takes getting shaken to the core to shift gears and redirect momentum. Sometimes we need to plant, nurture, and water something different and watch that grow when the consequence of continuing to live half-heartedly becomes too great.

Deciding to make a change requires a conscious pivoting of our mindsets. A choice to move forward and see the beauty in life again. A choice to search for the potential in the challenge and ultimately work to find ourselves again. If we don't keep hold, circumstances can contort us into unrecognizable people. Finding our way back to a better version of ourselves is possible, one with greater knowledge of the human experience, greater emotional depth and understanding, and a sense of peace that we are making the best of our current circumstances. Life is about becoming – becoming who we are made to be. We are all in the process of becoming. It's not just in the easy, free-flowing times of life, but more importantly, in deeply challenging times.

When life is smooth, and we aren't challenged, it's easy to become complacent. The trials we face bring about the meaning and the potential for significant impact when we use the lessons to better ourselves and support others. There is value and importance in times of struggle when we look for it. There lies the potential for greater depth, a strengthened character, identification of meaningful priorities, and enhancing one's resilience. Taking time to reflect in the face of pain and suffering can provide meaning.

Every fictional superhero has a tragic backstory; by overcoming adversity, they realize their potential. Hardship has the power to shape us into much better versions of ourselves if we are open to exploring it. It works the other way too. Many superhero villains and real-life jaded and angry people are that way as they succumb to their adversity and allow the roots of bitterness and envy to take hold of their hearts. We are faced with this choice, and the decision has the potential to change the rest of our lives.

Experiencing infertility allowed me to connect with others facing infertility in a meaningful way. Feeling overwhelmed by my circumstances allowed me to sit with the discomfort of other people feeling overwhelmed by their circumstances. Not knowing how I would come out the other end of the pain allows me to feel comfortable with others who are unsure of how their story will end. Relating to one another is the essence of a relationship. There is so much to learn in these challenging times. A deeper understanding of ourselves through self-reflection and building a greater capacity for empathy towards other people are some of the more positive things that have come from this experience of infertility. I hope you can find your version of this on your journey. I hope you become your version of a superhero.

Thoughts on Growth

While in high school, I felt ready and excited to move on to university by about Grade 11. While in university, I thought I was prepared to move to post-secondary education to get closer to my career. While in naturopathic medical school, I felt ready to complete all of the requirements necessary to live in the "real world" with a real job. It's natural to anticipate the next step and seek the progress of reaching the next stop along your path. However, there is growth and purpose in the waiting during the current stage we find ourselves in. Those final high school years are required for development and maturity that we draw on during the university years, or whatever stage is to follow. Those university years were needed to develop the independence, capacity, and intrinsic motivation required for the next season life had in store for me. For myself, those grueling years of naturopathic medical school were needed to become the ND I am today.

One foot must come before the other to prepare for the path ahead. That is where significant growth happens – the process of each step along the way, in the grinding times, in the slowing-down times, and in the hard work of the task at hand. Growth is not just achieving the next step. It's in the journeying through. Robert Holden says, "Beware of destination addiction. Destination addiction is the preoccupation with the idea that happiness is in the next place, the next job, and with the next partner. Until you give up the idea that happiness is somewhere else, it will never be where you are."[8]

Frustration can become a constant companion when we aren't progressing and moving forward. One summer, we decided to plant a vegetable garden. We built a raised garden bed and started researching vegetable and soil options. I went to a local organic farm to purchase the recommended soil combination and chose our seeds. What I hadn't realized at the time was how therapeutic the process of planting seeds and watching them grow would be for me. I would water the garden and check on the growth of these tiny seeds every day, and bit by bit, little by little, the stronger they grew. The process became almost meditative.

Each day I could see the result of a day of full sun, or a good heavy rain, and tending to the weeds to support the growing environment. This daily practice of nurturing, managing, and caring for these growing plants helped pacify the internal desire to nurture. It supported my intrinsic desire to help things grow, and it made me feel so great to be able to feed ourselves healthy vegetables. The "vegetables of my labor" was a metaphor for that time in life. It helped me redirect the emotional pain and stress of infertility to focus on something that brought me joy. All while trying something new and investing energy into something that would result in growth. You never know. Other areas of your life outside of infertility can help positively influence your experience as you navigate through it.

We can't fast-forward this season, can't go around, under or over it. With intentionality, we can find our best way through it. I urge you to find something that you can work towards as a short-term goal. Maybe it involves trying new recipes, investing time in a charitable initiative, or learning a new artistic skill. I know someone who went through infertility and chose to go to a teacher's college, completely changing her career course. Someone else went to medical school and became a doctor during their infertility journey. We never know what opportunities you may be prompted to explore or what direction your life may go as a result.

There is a benefit in continuing to move forward and putting energy into investing in the future. It's even better when you focus on an area within greater control. Spend time contemplating what this might be for you, big or small. It releases some of the pressure that builds as time goes on.

Questions:

1. What area in your life do you want to foster growth?
2. What areas are you working on growing in your life?
3. What lessons can you draw from your current challenges?
4. Looking back at yourself before beginning treatment,

what are three ways you have changed for the better?

5. What is one way you can see this journey positively molding you? What are three things you can do to encourage this change?

LIE #9: SUCCESS IS A POSITIVE PREGNANCY TEST

A great dichotomy exists when we view infertility as success and failure. This rigid way of thinking can make us stumble. The infertility experience lends itself to viewing things as black or white. Did the treatment work? Did the treatment fail? Did the protocol result in the hormonal changes expected? Did it not? Beta testing has a positive or negative result. The process and structure of the medical infertility experience allow for two outcomes: success or failure, pass or fail, and these are the words used to describe these scenarios. The process funnels you into this rigid mindset where you either get the checkmark or the big red X. But in the reality of life, there are other possibilities and directions. It's not so clear-cut.

For those who are early on or supporting someone along this journey, you may not understand the process of treatments or assessment for infertility. A very generalized overview may involve an assessment with bloodwork for hormonal analysis (I believe my initial blood test involved 25 vials of blood being taken) and a sperm analysis and basic bloodwork for the male partner. Progressing from there consists of a series of ultrasounds and blood tests at specific times in the female menstrual cycle to evaluate hormone changes and follicle growth to establish the timing of ovulation and treatments. Further actions include intervening with specific drugs at particular times of the cycle to manipulate the hormones according to the potential concerns and tracking the cycle with pelvic ultrasounds. Intrauterine insemination (IUI) and in vitro fertilization (IVF) are the medical interventions often used to address infertility and increase the chances of pregnancy.

Several medical appointments are required per week during a treatment cycle, with precisely timed hormone treatments, oral medications, injections, and/or vaginal suppositories. The treatments run your life as they are precisely timed and based on uncontrolled factors learned as you go through the treatments. Each day you learn what the next day may bring. The combination of invasive procedures, hormones that often interfere with mood and energy, and the uncertainty of the outcome of this time/ energy/financial investment leads to a spiraling season in one's life.

You have more power and ownership in the definition of success than the experience of infertility leads you to believe. A simple test does not. People define success in many different ways: accumulating material possessions and having the latest gadget, sporting a trendy wardrobe, owning an upscale house, driving a fancy car, reaching an athletic accomplishment, or honing certain character traits. Our experiences, upbringing, and view of the world determine the parameters in place that influence how we set out to define success. Fertility clinics have statistics on how well their techniques and procedures perform, resulting in a healthy pregnancy and live birth rate, a determining success rate.

Infertility forced me to acknowledge my rigid definition of success at that time in my journey. For me, it was pass or fail, as the system's structure defines it. Several treatment cycles without a successful pregnancy were undoubtedly discouraging, and it made me feel like a failure. Growing up, I felt a running race was either won or lost. The accolade was achieved, or it wasn't. High standards with a razor-thin margin for error often led to unrealistic expectations of myself. When we focus on the outcome rather than the process, we can lose a lot along the way.

A stiff, rigid outlook leaves you bruised when things fall apart.

There is flexibility and softness required to help adapt, maneuver, learn, and navigate new directions. Fertility treatments were a natural progression after being pregnant and miscarrying at the start of our family-building journey. The last embryo implanted was at the end of that era.

My husband and I discussed expanding our family through adoption; it had always been part of our plan. With the province's regulations regarding being unable to adopt while trying to conceive, we were now at the stage to go back to the idea of adoption and seek out the following steps on that journey. Adoption has always been a step we planned to take, and the time had come to start the process.

This season of life has allowed me to see the advantage of redefining these thought patterns and the benefits of a flexible mindset. There are no two human beings alike, so it would not make sense to have a singular definition of success in any form. When life is observed through a rigid mindset, the emotional turmoil that follows is equally intense. It's stressful to stay in the lines, which is not the purpose of this life. We are familiar with the month-to-month anticipation of fulfilling hopes and dreams, followed by the crash of those dreams not coming true. I started viewing each month as a month closer to learning how our family would come to be. How it was meant to be, and removing this pass/fail mentality. I began learning to open myself up to changing timelines and engage in life more fully in the present. We worked towards our family, and time would tell how that would play out.

This process of setting and working toward goals involves engaging in something greater than ourselves. The goal is less important when compared to the meaning we attach to these goals.

The timing of our adoption process aligned with us being matched with our son Pete, which is incredible to think about. He was always part of our family plan, but we didn't know that for many years along the way. We built our family through our love for each other and our love for our son, even before he was born. Life is not black and white; family planning is not black and white. Success is in the process and learning along the way.

I would describe my experience of infertility as incredibly successful; personal growth and change have taken place through the process. Developing a greater self-awareness, more profound love and respect in our marriage, and identifying our hopes and dreams at the core; to have a family. I bet if you are reading this, it may feel a little far-fetched – obnoxious, even. I can relate to that, as I have spent many years struggling through this myself. I've been at the social events of people announcing their pregnancies, putting on a face of happiness while choking back a breakdown. It's understandable that even reading about us being matched with our son may elicit a visceral response in you. That makes sense. You are desperate for your story to reach a happy ending too. I've needed breathers from hearing others' good news stories also. Take the time you need.

If success is a happy family, I would kindly offer that you don't want to settle for feeling miserable while waiting for that. Feel it, evaluate it for what that means for you, just don't camp out there for the long haul. Understand the broader picture of what adjusting your definition can offer you. Find that contentment in your current circumstances while you work towards what your family may become.

We built our family through international adoption. Our son was meant to be in our family, and we were meant to be his parents. The extra time we had ended up being an opportunity to build up even more love and hopeful anticipation for what our future family would come to be.

You may find that your family comes to be in the way you imagined, maybe just on a different timeline. You may find that your entire view shifts, and you start to see your world in a totally new way. I think the key is remaining teachable and open to the process, understanding that there is more than one way to build your family, and the way that lines up for you is meant for you. You are a family now. Life is not black and white; family planning isn't either. Take inventory of how you define success for yourself to offer yourself some emotional flexibility during this time.

Questions:

1. What are some of your biggest successes? What makes them a win for you?
2. Have you had any situations that you defined as failures in the past that have become learning opportunities?
3. How have you learned from a previous "failure"?
4. What would it look like if you removed a success/fail mindset towards your infertility journey?

LIE #10: WE MUST ALWAYS WORK HARDER

Addressing infertility demands a certain level of grit. Persistence is required to take continuous action, and momentum builds as time, energy, and a sense of urgency build. Pushing through challenges can be a double-edged sword, and the strength required to keep fighting can be the same weakness that ignores personal needs at the expense of the fight.

When a challenge comes up, it makes sense to create a plan and overcome it. That's a natural response. Sustained stress draws on our resources and causes drain. Looking back on the hard times that I've faced in my life, it's easy to see that pushing through has been a default setting. We excel at the very things that can become our biggest downfalls when swinging too far in the other direction. Some of the kindest people I know can very easily overextend themselves to the detriment of their health. The most productive people I know can get into zones where they can't pause their work struggle to be in the moment and engage in meaningful connections.

Striking a balance is what it's all about.

Initially, pushing through the challenges of infertility can be incredibly helpful. With each obstacle, you can experience a quick dusting off and regrouping to prepare to tackle the next one – battle mode activated. This allows us to get through many tough things and continue to function. There was one day that I rushed to put my name on the waitlist at the ultrasound clinic (first-come, first-served) at our local hospital, drove to my clinic office to see a couple of patients, returning for the ultrasound just as my name was called up, and then back to work for the rest of the day.

Everything timed down to the minute. Efficient? Maybe. Sustainable? Not at all.

Rushing fuels anxiety and is an indication of pushing past the limits. Razor-thin margins only look great in retrospect when reviewing the tasks that are now complete. We are robbed of engaging in life in the moment, which is life as we know it. We get caught up in keeping up with these unrealistic demands. I'm sure you've faced your fair share of difficult situations and leveled up to the challenges this season has brought to you in the name of getting by and pushing through. Over time, infertility taught me the importance of regularly tending to my emotional well-being, which didn't come naturally while this battle mode was activated.

Adrenaline is a beautiful thing; it's life-saving, actually. When there is a threat, like a wild animal in your room, our adrenaline is life-saving as this automatic stress response allows us to think clearly, and it primes our bodies to react and run away or fight off the animal. Our heart beats faster, our breathing rate increases, our blood flows to our skeletal muscles, and our pupils dilate to give us the best chances of survival. All systems go to deal most efficiently with the threat at hand. The challenge comes when our body misinterprets situations like the scheduling conflicts of infertility treatments, the urgent changes to a treatment protocol, or the anticipation of a test result, as the same threat as a dangerous animal. While feeling stressed in these situations is valid, the sustained impact of consistently being on high alert has damaging long-term consequences and is a fast-track ticket to burnout.

While pushing through infertility, ignoring our emotional needs damages our physical and emotional health.

My emotions' impact on my health and well-being wasn't apparent while I was in the thick of this journey. Our body and mind being intimately connected are now conversations I have with my patients every day. Unfelt emotions that are unexpressed and untended drain us. The stress lingers in our bodies. Being "tough" and pushing through the pain is not always helpful, as there are too many big feelings involved, and our bodies keep the score. Unfelt emotions linger, and they get bigger and bigger in time. As it turns out, being emotionally aware and attuned is an incredible strength. Allowing ourselves to process and feel in real-time is a skill that makes this process smoother.

After completing our treatments, I started reading books on infertility. Much of my learning was hindsight, and this reading confirmed that unfelt and undealt with emotions have a significant impact. The book *"Experiencing Infertility"* by Peoples and Rovner Ferguson[9] likened the stress of infertility to someone going through a diagnosis of cancer or HIV. That secretive, perceived shameful experience of mine was a bottled-up land mine. Reading this brought so much relief and validation and acknowledged my emotional pain. It confirmed that my intense feelings were real, expected, and in line with the severity of the situation. I wish I knew then what I know now.

The experience of infertility is massive, and it's not something to face in a sustained fighting position.

Settle in, look around you, feel the feelings coming up as you navigate through. It's a lot, and no wonder this experience brings about feelings that have never been felt before.

Peoples and Rovner Ferguson[9] discussed infertility as a standalone risk factor for anxiety and depression. Understanding this now, both personally and professionally, I can identify early signs of these coming up with my patients. What we need in times like this is the courage and strength to offer ourselves compassion at a greater level than the brute force of continuously jumping over the hurdles, one after another. Emotional awareness and grit is an act of courage and demonstrable strength. Despite infertility being so common, the emotional toll it takes can be extraordinary. Everyday experiences don't necessitate glossing over the impact. Acknowledge the feelings; all feelings are valid.

When I started medicated cycles, the medical professional in me wanted to know every detail of the treatment protocol, the intended purpose, duration, and makeup of the medications. I wanted to be primed and ready to tackle this infertility process. It began by looking up the drugs, their impact on the body, their intended use, the benefits and potential side effects, and where they came from. Super cool, right? It was fascinating and informative and satisfied my desire to feel a sense of control over the treatment plan. Then I got to Ovidrel. As I was researching, I came across this excerpt, "The production process involves expansion of genetically modified Chinese Hamster Ovary (CHO) cells..."[10] I immediately burst into tears. You don't have to be an ND to have feelings about the idea of these CHO cells being injected into your body.

The overwhelming nature of the situation and the bizarre medication origin left me in tears giving myself these injections. The stress of the potential risks and consequences of taking the medications were aggravated by feeling handcuffed to the treatment protocols I was choosing to pursue. None of it felt comfortable, and my joy was drained while injecting myself with the hope of a family. I pushed through. I bypassed my feelings by rationalizing our choice and the privilege we had to access advanced medicine at this time in history and the resources we had access to. We can feel grateful and uncertain at the same time. We can acknowledge our desire to control more in a season where things feel out of control. The work comes in releasing and surrendering.

Some people may find learning about the details of the treatment plan to be empowering and helpful, easing anxieties about the unknown. For myself, having too much information or knowing too much was causing stress because it led to overthinking and catastrophizing thoughts during this vulnerable time. By identifying components of the process that contribute to feeling overwhelmed, we can create boundaries to help manage them. We can stop researching things that add to the stress and change nothing about the action plan. We can remove triggering people on our social feed. Some can change work hours to reduce the strain on timing appointments. Perhaps some of you reading this have remnants of genetically modified Chinese hamster ovary cells in your body too. Welcome to the club. It is evidence of the things we do in the name of love and the hope of a family.

Shifting my desire for complete control to sharing that load with my team of trusted medical professionals was a helpful decision and necessary to manage the stress I was adding to the situation. Conscious mindset shifts are required through emotionally taxing times. The reality was that my pharmacist, who filled my prescription, didn't even know where Ovidrel came from. At this time, I intentionally chose to free my mind from this chatter once the decision to take it was made. Addressing uncomfortable situations as they arise helps to manage emotions longer term. A great stress-reducing strategy is acknowledging what we can and can't control. Make a plan for what can be controlled and release the outcome of what can't be controlled. Allow yourselves to feel your emotions through the process as they unfold. Do a little, feel a little, as a wise friend once shared with me. Then, do a little more, and then feel a little more.

"Pushing through" delayed self-compassion at a time when I could have used it most. When we learn to identify our feelings as they come up, learn about our triggers, and make changes to support our emotional well-being along the way, this is when we can create positive change. This is a sign of strength, a tool we can use to soften the process. We need to cushion ourselves with compassion rather than armoring up with a hard outer shell during our preparations for battle. With this as my motto, I would have done things differently. I hope you can give yourself the space to be human in this process.

A typical stress trigger is the last-minute changing of plans and the uncertain scheduling of infertility treatments. For a few years, I straddled the pressure of showing up for my patients and showing up for myself with my fertility treatments. There were many times when showing up for myself had to take precedence, which led to last-minute scheduling changes at work. This was incredibly stressful and piled on the feeling of not being my best self in multiple areas of life. It was easy to internalize the notion that I was disappointing others. My business had been my "baby" through these years, an area to invest my energy and time that felt meaningful and valuable. Not being able to predict when to go for bloodwork or ultrasounds because each appointment provided information for the next was stressful. My goodness, the not knowing runs so deep in this struggle.

There was no way around the schedule interruptions, yet I worried the same every day that involved a change in my schedule. Look for patterns of pain. Once I became aware that I was caught up in this cycle of feeling anxious every time I had to cancel patients, it became clear that something had to change. It wasn't a situation that involved fighting through it and expecting things to change. This situation caught my attention enough to tune in to my needs, make a change, and soften the experience and expectations of myself moving forward.

Specific shifts of thinking had to take place. It involved reminding myself that these tests were a non-negotiable component of the treatment. I chose to put my hope for a family as my top priority, above my career, for this season. While simply saying these things to myself didn't miraculously take the stress away, it did help to regroup when the familiar discomfort would arise around this known trigger. Continuing to battle my way through the unsettled feelings would have only made things worse, or at best, I consistently felt upset and stressed each time I needed to cancel an appointment. I reminded myself regularly that my priorities supported the release of these emotions in a situation that was out of my control. Anxiety could have been a companion with every interrupted day; however, accepting and adjusting my expectations during this season allowed me to release the guilt attached to changing plans.

When we tune into our emotions, we can use them as a guide. Stop and reflect regularly to allow space and grace for yourself and those around you. We can't be everything to everyone, especially during this time. Sometimes we have to pull back in certain areas to pour into areas demanding more attention. Giving yourself a bit of space and time to pay attention to these patterns of emotions can allow greater insight into your specific needs. Adjusting to the detours of life can't quickly happen when living life in fast-forward. Sometimes we need to push forward, and other times it's wise and helpful to pull back to regroup and reassess. At times we lean in, and other times we lean out. We must mindfully use that healthy margin to process and implement necessary changes. The grueling and challenging bits of life lead us to the juicy center of ourselves and our capacity to overcome. We simply can't get there if we never allow ourselves to reflect.

What was once an intensely stressful period is now something I can look back on with knowledge of how much I've grown from it all. I find myself joking about the funny nuances of the wild rollercoaster of it all. Life is complicated and challenging. Sometimes we feel like we're barely holding on, and other times we coast along feeling settled and relaxed. Bringing awareness to our emotional health along the journey and tending to these needs allow us to take care of ourselves along the way.

The irony in facing this challenging season is the thought that I leveled up and pushed through the physical process, thinking that was a strength of mine. Still, in reality, it has taken a lot more courage to acknowledge the emotional pain in the process. Feeling pain is a courageous act that allows us to ultimately work through it. Work towards creating more margin in your days and in your life to allow for the space needed to understand your own needs and make breathing room for the twists and turns that inevitably occur. Surrendering what cannot be controlled and creating space for feeling through it is the way forward.

L.R. Knost says so beautifully, "life is amazing. And then it's awful. And then it's amazing again. And in between the amazing and awful it's ordinary and mundane and routine. Breathe in the amazing, hold on through the awful, and relax and exhale during the ordinary. That's just living a heartbreaking, soul-healing, amazing, awful, ordinary life. And it's breathtakingly beautiful."[11]

Questions:

1. Do you find yourself "pushing through" in this season of life? How does that feel?
2. What physical sensations come up when you are feeling acutely stressed? Pay attention the next time you feel stressed and tune in to how your body feels. This can be used as a cue to highlight in the future.
3. What are three ways you can engage in self-compassion? Some of my favorites are taking an Epsom salt bath at the end of the day, carving out time in the day to be in nature, and being realistic with the expectations I place on myself.

BOUNDARIES

FINDING PURPOSE IN THE ROUGH SEASONS

The experience of living through the rough, painful, and unsettling season that infertility brings can reveal many new opportunities. These rough seasons usher in growth opportunities and chances to build self-awareness, allowing us to exercise self-compassion and empathy.

Tough experiences can be reframed as productive struggles if we are willing and open. Learning and growth don't happen when things are easy; remaining easy and safe keeps you firmly planted just as you are. If you have ever worked hard to learn a new skill, you know that pushing yourself to move just beyond that comfort zone or that space where things are easy moves you into that place where significant gains can happen. As we allow ourselves to reframe struggles as a productive space, we notice more clearly the things that overcoming these lies is pushing us to learn.

More importantly, perhaps, when we recognize that this rough season is one of productive struggle, it allows us to move well beyond the stagnant zone that's all too comfortable to inhabit.

Rough Seasons Teach Us About Compassion

Brené Brown's words capture the essence of compassion so beautifully: "Don't look away. Don't look down. Don't pretend not to see hurt. Look people in the eye. Even when their pain is overwhelming. And when you're hurting and in pain, find the people who can look you in the eye."[12]

Infertility was not the first rough season in my life, and it won't be the last. Early in university, my mom was on a slow and steady decline in her physical and cognitive health. Her condition was unknown at the time. It affected her memory, cognition, coordination, and strength. Looking back, it started out as comical moments. She would ask us where her fork was during dinner when she was holding it in her hand. We would laugh and poke fun until we quickly realized that it wasn't funny. It was something much more severe than a momentary lapse in judgment. This continued to worsen over the next few years, at which time her doctor recommended experimental chemotherapy be administered in the cerebrospinal fluid. I wasn't medically trained when her health began to fail, and the details of her health decline weren't clear to me, other than I knew it was a big deal and my mom was not okay.

In the earlier stages of her decline, I remember learning about nutrition and how food impacted the body. I would call her from a payphone in the University of Guelph library to tell her what she needed to eat to help her memory and health. When her chemotherapy treatments began, I lived in Toronto with my aunt and uncle (my mother's brother) to become a naturopathic doctor during my first year of school. My mom was three weeks into her chemotherapy protocol when she suffered a seizure in the night, leaving her in a coma that she would ultimately never recover from.

Receiving that phone call on my lunch break at school is permanently imprinted in my brain. I walked into a stairwell so I could hear my dad speak. Once I listened to what he said, I physically collapsed on the floor from the shock of this horrifying news. Three weeks after her seizure, she passed away. While her health was declining, I felt like I was free-falling off a cliff into a completely unexpected situation. There is no preparation for this level of grief. Losing my mother at the impressionable age of 21 was a devastation that forever changed me. I feel things deeper. I care for others more intensely. My compassion and empathy towards those suffering can sometimes be painful, knowing the depth of such pain myself. The intensity of grief is a consequence of loving and being loved deeply. We can grow in times of suffering.

Without walking this journey of deep grief, I would not have a reference point for deep suffering. Without feeling this deep pain personally, I would not understand the pain of others. Experience brings perspective, and I couldn't understand grief before experiencing it myself. We don't choose to suffer, and none of us ever would. It's easy to wallow in suffering, and it's painfully hard to choose to learn and grow in times of suffering, but the suffering itself is consistent across both options.

I share this story with you not to elicit sympathy but share that even in *life's most painful experiences*, we can learn valuable lessons that influence our lives. It took me the better part of a decade to extract anything positive from this particular season of profound grief. Growth and learning don't follow a linear timeline with our grief and suffering; however, the capacity is there, and we can learn when we are ready.

We aren't meant to journey through our struggles alone. We are all in this life together, doing the best we can with the cards we've been dealt. Being honest about our struggles allows for authentic relationships. Great relationships are built on people being their true, broken selves and accepting this is solidified by experiencing this connection. Are you struggling too? Oh, your life isn't perfect either? This offers such tremendous relief. Surface living is an existence. Authenticity supports genuinely living. The people who mean the most to us are the ones who are invested in your answer when asking how you are. These people celebrate during the high moments and support you during the low moments. We struggle and celebrate together. We share the load to lighten the burden. Life's short, and it's too exhausting to be anything but true to ourselves. Whether facing infertility, family struggles, relationship challenges, losses, uncertainty, fears, or failures, life is full of challenges. Life is more manageable when we aren't hiding our insecurities and assumed inadequacies. We are all in it together.

There is value in finding meaning in pain. It seems wasteful and worthless to allow suffering to pass along without purpose. While this doesn't gloss over the loss or pain, it provides insight that can be life-giving. Hard things happen in life and can have purpose and meaning when given space and time to process. This helps to make sense of this world. Life can be excruciatingly painful, and the depths of despair so vast. Everyone is finding their own way and doing the best they can. We can't always make sense of these challenges, but there can be meaning despite not understanding the logic or accepting reality.

When my mom passed away, all I felt about it was a spectrum of negative emotions. It was too painful to fully feel the emotional loss, let alone find anything I could accept as meaningful among all the hurt. All I could see was that I had to live my life without my mom and all of the losses that were still to come within that reality. It was the deep grief of being a motherless daughter. It wasn't until years later that I could see in myself the ability to connect with others in their suffering; I could do so in a way that people could feel seen. I could offer an exchange of "I've been shattered and built back up again too." Previous to this experience – as a happy-go-lucky individual whose life always showed up rose-colored – I didn't have the personal experience to feel or connect with others experiencing pain or hardship in this way. There was no context. We can grow from pain.

We will have many more battles to face in this life, this is for sure. May we continue to choose learning and growth as we fight and feel our way through it. The opposite of this allows cynicism to infiltrate, and the world doesn't need any more of that. Choose purpose, meaning and joy.

BOUNDARIES WITH
YOUR TIME

Infertility may require us to change boundaries in various aspects of our lives. It can take specific attention in multiple areas of your life to help identify what a healthy version will look like to support your experience through it. This may be a new topic to discover or an area requiring greater awareness at this time. Boundaries may not be a topic that has required much thought in the past, and I hadn't put much thought into my boundaries until I had to.

It started becoming more clear when my expectations extended beyond my capacity. There was a lot of self-talk that involved thoughts like, "I *should* do the same amount of work in addition to the fertility treatments, regardless of what my body and mind can accomplish." "Should-ing" is exhausting. Have you noticed that? I *should* go to this event. I *should* connect with this friend. I *should* help with this event. Identifying when the "should-ing" starts to take over has become an essential tool to use as a cue to step back from the situation and see what is best. If we aren't careful, we can "should" our way through life and not live it on purpose, for *our* purpose.

Our energy has limits. The emotional energy exerted through treatment alone is grounds for exhaustion, not to mention the necessities of work, household responsibilities, volunteer commitments, or other additional responsibilities. Time is precious and non-renewable. Preserving and conserving energy wherever possible is needed for staying power in the journey. Simple changes can make a big difference. One baby shower is enough to throw anyone off their infertility game and put a damper on an entire weekend. You don't need to be a hero or please everyone around you. You are a human being, so give yourself permission to say no. When a "yes" to someone else is saying a loud "no" to yourself, that's where things become damaging if it becomes a habit. Slow down your "yes" game to give yourself time to reflect on how you are spending your precious gift of time. Is it an accurate reflection of the direction you want to move forward in – towards better health and wellness or exhaustion and burnout? Your answer is the summation of your individual choices.

Personal boundaries are set by ourselves or default to what others ask of us. Healthy boundaries create healthier relationships. Overextending ourselves to meet the demands of others may come at the expense of our physical and mental well-being. Lack of boundary setting will leave us vulnerable to the sway of what others ask of us. When we overextend ourselves, we're not able to show up as the people we need to be for our loved ones, to connect with family and friends in a valuable way, and we can't be the person we need to be for ourselves.

Unhealthy boundaries lead to resentment towards people we offer help to, and there is no one to blame but ourselves for this. Being the "yes" person and subsequently harboring resentment will hurt ourselves and our relationships. Some boundaries require rigid and firm structure, while others are fluid, as they shift with changing seasons, circumstances, and capacities.

Sometimes we have to say no when we otherwise would have said yes. There may be times that require declining an invitation to a baby shower or a children's birthday party. I skipped out on my fair share and felt totally fine with sending a present in place of my presence. The sentiment remains, but we take care of our mental health in the process. This was a personal boundary that I needed to set for myself, and no one else could do it for me. There are other times when I accepted these invitations or hosted parties myself. This changed throughout my fertility experience.

Boundaries and guilt are familiar companions. Guilt and negative thoughts can dictate our lives if we don't interject. Don't let them creep in and force you to do something you don't have the emotional capacity for. When talking to yourself in "shoulds," step back and re-evaluate if you need to torment yourself or if the people around you who love you will be glad that you are protecting yourself, even if they can't fully understand at the moment.

Passing on an invitation may be better than an awkward outburst of emotions in the middle of a room full of people you barely know (or wasting energy that you don't have on all the feelings that it will stir up). We only have so much energy, and we must be wise with how and when we exert ourselves.

I wasn't fully aware of the emotional toll of infertility until it was over. While being in it, it's hard to comprehend and feel its impact fully. I suggest you offer yourself a little space to evaluate what feels suitable for you and give yourself more buffer than you think you need.

Skipping events may honor your boundaries at some points of the journey, while at other times, your capacity may allow for your attendance. My two older sisters were expecting at the same time around the start of my infertility treatments. It was a demanding and overwhelming time as I was coming to terms with my reality. Hosting a double baby shower for them was a personal choice to support my sisters in their joy and excitement and being the sister I wanted to be for them. It was intentional and difficult, and it was the right decision. Missing out on many friends' baby showers was also my reality and the right decision at the time.

That's where the fluidity of boundaries comes in. There aren't any hard and fast rules. You may love to surround yourself with babies and families and celebrations of new life. If so, that's awesome! Embrace it and enjoy it. It is certainly worth celebrating. If it's not, there is nothing wrong with you. It is normal to have difficulty separating the emotional complexity of pure joy and happiness for others while feeling painfully raw and distraught about your own childlessness. Do what you need to do when you need to do it. One week you may accept an invite to the party. You may need to create space from your friends with kids the following week. It's okay. There is no rubric to follow during this time. Let yourself feel these feelings and process them while honoring your needs as you decide. Some people will understand, and others won't. They don't have to. Without having the experience of infertility, it's nearly impossible to fully appreciate its complexities. Take the time to be sure that you understand and honor yourself.

Questions:

1. What activities do you find draining?
2. What activities bring you energy?
3. Critically evaluate your commitments and how they make you feel before, during and afterward. Let this help determine the best use of your time and resources.

BOUNDARIES FOR YOUR TREATMENT

As treatments progress over time, there are difficult decisions to make. How long do you continue with treatments? What types of treatments are you (and your partner) okay with? How much can you handle emotionally? When is enough really enough? How are long-term finances impacted by the following steps, and is this even feasible? These answers are as unique as our fingerprints.

The challenge with so many decisions we face at each step of the journey is that the answers can't be known until each decision is met explicitly in real-time. The facts and feelings on various issues of future events aren't clear, and they can't be clear. It's best to identify when you are trying to make a future decision and leave those decisions for the future.

I remember talking with Erik and mentioning that we would never do IVF when we knew some friends were going through it. We hadn't even started trying to conceive at this point; therefore, we didn't have the information to make that judgment call. We didn't know, it wasn't our decision to make at the time, and we had no idea what was involved until it became our reality.

We can't know what we don't know, and spending time and energy on future decisions turns out to be a waste of both precious resources. Catch yourself if you find yourself circling around "what if" scenarios, and remind yourself that it's a future decision that isn't meant for the present. There are enough decisions and items to process day-to-day; carrying your future load is too heavy. Keeping your mind and decisions focused on your current reality keeps future worries off the shoulders of your current circumstance.

Concluding that the infertility treatment road has ended is an emotionally-charged decision. There are no guidelines for this, and no one can decide for you. Everyone's "done" will look different. For some, it may be a pregnancy. For others, it will be when a biological clock rings the alarm, and others may decide that it's just time to be done. Some conclude the journey as soon as medical intervention is required, once the IUI option is exhausted, the need for a non-biological embryo, or when finances dictate that moving forward is no longer an option.

Whatever "done" looks like, there isn't a concrete formula to organize your thought process on the matter. It involves being true to yourself and what you (and your partner) are prepared for and decide. Personally, being "done" smacked me across the face. Being done for you may be a silent whisper of your body saying, "I'm tired. I need to rest." When we stay connected to our needs throughout the journey, we can keep tabs on our emotional reserves and capacity. There won't always be a clear, confident answer to indicate when you may be done. It doesn't have to make sense. It doesn't have to be justified. Your decision should honor where you are and what is suitable for you. No one else around you has to agree with your decision. This may be one of the most challenging personal decisions you and your partner make. Take the time you need – trust yourself, and be true to yourself.

After two rounds of IVF and several embryo transfers, my body and mind were completely finished. When we began IVF, we didn't know that we would complete two rounds of it, and we didn't know that we would even do IVF in the first place until that was the next step forward. I think of being younger and asking, "How do you know when you're in love?" The typical response was, "When you know, you know." There is no context to knowing until you're in it.

Understanding what's next or how being "done" feels is similar. There are fewer butterflies and googly eyes, but deep down, you *know* or in some circumstances, it is spelled out. When you're giving yourself the space to tune in with your sense of understanding, you will know when it is time to be finished with this step of the journey. While it was evident to me, it may not be as straightforward for others. For some, it may seem vague, uncertain, without absolutes to clearly mark out a path, or clouded with complexities when experiencing mismatched thoughts with your partner. No one can tell you when enough is enough. Or when you've gone as far as you are meant to go. They can't tell you the outcome of any decision or when it's time to switch gears. Certainty is not a component of infertility. Each experience we go through helps prepare us for what we may face next. And so, the story of life goes. One challenge builds resilience and the capacity to meet the next. You can never know how you'll feel about the next challenge until you are staring it in the eyes. No one else can tell you what is right for you. It's impossible to know what you'll think or feel about a future step before its natural timing.

Levels of certainty change as information and experiences change. Frankly, uncertainty is one of the most significant challenges faced by infertility. There was a time when I felt confident that one round of IVF, which involved four embryo transfers, would be the only round we ever did. Then we entered a new reality that we hadn't faced before. There is no systematic way to decide what is right for you. For us, we booked a follow-up appointment with our reproductive endocrinologist to discuss what had transpired and bring a sense of closure to this infertility intervention phase. After our appointment and a hopeful discussion with our specialist, it was strongly recommended that we meet with the clinic's fertility-focused ND, follow a new protocol for several months, and then try IVF again. That hope and plan led us on an intensive eight-month prep and subsequent round of IVF. I would never have expected to do a second round of IVF before this appointment. New information brought new decisions.

Being a patient was an intriguing and insightful experience. I prefer being the doctor and helping patients more than being one; however, it helped me understand how my patients feel when they struggle and need support. It takes courage to ask for help, and I think it is something to celebrate. That being said, despite being initially closed off to the idea of doing a second round of IVF, when we were faced with this new information, we made a different choice.

Decisions can only be made in real-time; preparing for future decisions is a drain on limited energy.

Planning and preparing ahead of time is futile and exhausting. As tempting as it is, it merely falsely pacifies the fear of the unknown and the uncertainty surrounding the experience by offering a taste of control. It's a waste of precious energy and stimulates worry. While the decision-making process itself doesn't follow a rubric, a routine check-in with yourself (and your partner) can be a beneficial practice.

Keeping in tune with your capacity, feelings, and thoughts as each partner navigate their own experience can help the partnership navigate together instead of separately if this is a partnered decision.

Pre-determining your potential future steps causes anxiety and worry when, in fact, those circumstances may never be yours to ever worry about. A full mind in a looped strategizing mode is not a healthy mind. Give yourself space and allow for mental wiggle room. Take a deep breath. Trust yourself and keep yourself in the current stage of your struggle. This load is heavy enough. Instead, redirect future thoughts and save them for when/if it becomes your reality. Today has enough worries of its own.

Our second IVF experience was a carbon copy of the first. We ended up with the same number of embryos to implant, with similar quality and the same result. We were able to implant two embryos simultaneously during the second experience, which allowed us to complete everything in two transfers instead of four. This lightened the load and duration of emotional strain.

I vividly remember the conversation with our specialist before our final transfer. Our doctor recommended a more intensive medication protocol for the best chance possible, knowing it would be our last transfer. He started describing this "long protocol" that would lead up to the transfer. "It will essentially put your body in a menopausal state, likely to include the associated side effects, including hot flashes, night sweats, insomnia, and mood disturbances." After about two minutes of introducing the protocol, my body and mind immediately resisted. I was done. This all had to stop. No month-long hormonal preparation. It had to end, and soon. I interrupted the doctor and thanked him for his commitment to my case and protocol, but I would not proceed. He knew I was done before we started the second round of IVF. So did my husband. This conversation left me with complete confidence in saying "no" and knowing that it was beyond what I was willing to sacrifice in addition to everything else I had already been through. I was met with compassion and understanding; my doctor heard me and respected my decision. We worked together to revamp the protocol in the least invasive, lowest dose of medication possible without sacrificing efficacy. I knew I was done and not meant to continue along this path.

After receiving our final negative pregnancy test, a wave of relief came over me. It had been such a battle for so long, and it was finally over. We fought a good fight, and now I could work on the final aspects of letting go. What may be seen as the most difficult part of an infertility journey was not for me. Grieving is a process that takes place with each passing month. At that moment, I could release myself from the expectations and pressure I had been putting on my body to perform. It was finished. There is no stone left unturned, no shortage of effort, time, energy, blood, sweat, or tears. We were empty, and it was time to move forward. It's exhausting to even think about that season.

Regardless of the decision, it's essential to take time and space to attune to what your body, relationship, and mind need. Establishing your treatment boundaries will help make tough decisions feel a bit easier, as you honor yourself rather than fighting against it/them. It was clear that my body was done, and my mind and heart were maxed out. It was an empowering experience to end this season by honoring what I knew was best, and it felt so right. Finishing the process on my terms was what I needed to do to heal from it all. When I knew, I *knew*. There are no guarantees this will be what you experience, and there are many unique factors that will make the decisions you make work best for you. When self-trust is profoundly challenged, it's a reconciling act to trust yourself. *Trust yourself.*

Right decisions don't always feel great. Making any decision can still leave a lot of tricky emotions to be sorted on the other end. The resolution process can often lead to feeling all the feelings that weren't felt or processed throughout the journey. It's a lot. Your mental headspace may need time to re-calibrate and download the complexity of the circumstances you've been through. It is traumatic. There was a great relief in knowing that my body wouldn't have to go through any more treatments, yet there were still feelings of sadness that I had to process, and that was okay.

Time helps to process and integrate your infertility experience with your story.

BOUNDARIES WITH
COMMUNICATION

─────── ⁓⁓ ───────

Deciding what you communicate and who you communicate with about your journey and what you keep private is entirely personal. Whether or not you openly share with others, you will hear various thoughts and opinions on building your family.

It's critical to separate these comments that feel shaming, judgemental, prideful, and awkward from the intentions of the person speaking them. We can't control what people say or react to us, but what we share and how we react is up to us. A popular quote says, "Ships don't sink because of the water around them; ships sink because of the water that gets in them." Don't let what's happening around you weigh you down; the situation is heavy enough on its own. Take in what is uplifting, encouraging, and helpful, and release what's discouraging, harmful, and untrue.

It's helpful to keep in mind that people are saying things from their broken journeys or something they are personally working through. Someone who says, "It's okay to be selfish and not have children," might be struggling and overwhelmed in their parenting experience. Just as they do not know the depths of our story, we do not know the depths of theirs. If anything, these comments are great reminders for us not to judge others and to avoid assumptions.

To help give others the benefit of the doubt, and quite frankly, to avoid intense reactions or outbursts, I try to remember that most comments are sincerely meant to help and are spoken out of curiosity, concern, or at times complete ignorance. Many statements can come across as hurtful when emotions are running high. Sometimes we can only nod our head and move on from the comment, or it may be an opportunity to say what we need to speak at the moment to express ourselves and educate others. People do not understand the depth of the pain elicited by making comments such as "You're next!" when all of your siblings are having children, or "You better get going, time is running out!", or "Try this___, it helped my great aunt conceive", or "Just relax" (emotional outburst-worthy comment). These are all comments that I have received. I'm sure you can easily add this list with your own experiences. People can only draw from their experiences, so as well-meaning as they may be, they don't understand how unhelpful it is and how it can diminish and downplay all of the effort and energy that has gone into the process.

These situations may become an opportunity to challenge other people's comments. There are always two sides to the coin, and some people may speak from a place of judgment, misunderstanding, or even an outdated worldview. There is an opportunity for growth and challenging their intent behind the words spoken in this case.

If there is a non-negotiable subject that gets brought up, you may want to have a prepared statement to communicate your point at the moment effectively. Personally, the best time to reflect on these is during my drive home from these situations that leave me otherwise stunned at the moment: "If someone is being ignorant and rude, then I will reply with how I feel." "If someone is genuinely invested, I can kindly accept their response and move forward, trusting their intention was good."

My parents' fertility experience was far different from mine, as they could time out our due dates for exactly after harvest was complete in the fall. No joke, their track record is evident. All four of us girls have birthdays between Oct. 24 and Nov. 23, a season where focus could shift from the field to the home. My dad's experience with infertility exists within his farming career, when raising cattle growing up. It is logical to draw from our personal experience as a reference point when relating to others.

When cows couldn't conceive, they would modify their diet to optimize their body weight. When they were too heavy or too thin, this impacted fertility. So naturally, my dad equated my experience to that of a heifer, with the hope of helping me conceive. Not surprisingly, my circumstances didn't translate to a skinny cow needing plumping. His intentions were pure, and it's pretty funny to look back on, but it was not a comment to take in and weigh me down at the time.

In all honesty, I was taken back at that moment – it was upsetting – before reminding myself of his intentions. It all felt like an oversimplification of a more complex issue and undermined my knowledge and efforts. At the time, I had already been to specialists, had a bombardment of testing, and had many treatment options underway. Whenever anyone gave me suggestions on what to do to support my efforts, I felt inadequate. The vulnerability of the topic and being sensitive toward others' ideas on the matter had me in a fragile state to begin with. It makes sense that a loving dad wants to help his struggling daughter realize her dream of having a family. It makes sense that close friends would share anything they knew on the topic, or a family member wishing to help in any way possible. Sharing information, if there was even the slightest potential to help the situation with someone you care about, is a loving thing to do. When we keep in mind others' intentions, we can understand the context of their words.

These situations have made me more aware of how powerful words are and how critically important it is not to judge or make assumptions. We never know the whole story and don't know the silent struggles people face. We must not make assumptions and focus on using our words to build others up rather than question or project what we think others "should" be doing. In the same way, we must choose the words we take in and filter out those that are not helpful or kind.

At the start of our treatments, I created a boundary with friends and family, establishing that I would bring up anything on infertility when I needed support. If I needed to talk about something, I would, but otherwise, I requested that they don't bring it up. At certain times I asked *before* sharing what I needed to say that I needed more of a listening ear on a particular topic rather than advice or words of comfort to help loved ones prepare to listen rather than racking their brain for the right words to say. Setting the stage helped both parties continue healthy communication rather than resentment of unmet needs. Asking for what is needed is a helpful, fruitful practice. Quite honestly, needs can vary so much during this confusing time. It can be a difficult conversation to have, but it's a part of protecting that relationship when you set these boundaries.

It was a Friday around noon when I saw the last patient of the week. I was walking them out of the door when she asked/told me, "So when are you having kids? You better get going since you're not getting any younger!" It was shocking. We weren't even talking about anything remotely related to the subject. I kid you not. I was 27 years old, and her healthcare provider, no less. We had just learned that our sixth IUI did not result in a pregnancy, and I was heading home to process it all. Yeah, words sting. They cut deep, even though the speaker of those harsh words had *no idea* of the impact. Being "on" at work allowed me to press on and laugh off the misplaced comment at the moment. It wasn't funny. Times like this would change the trajectory of the rest of my day. My guess is that you've had experiences like this too. It can be incredibly painful. Emotions linger until they find a place to rest and work themselves out. It's so hard to manage the words of others, especially when they aren't people to whom you are going to divulge such personal information. It's crucial to release the words of people who don't know the whole story and don't influence your life.

The things that people say can't be controlled. They say too much, or they say too little. They say things that feel like a physical kick to the gut. People will rarely say exactly what you need to hear or at a time you want to listen to it. When someone has never faced infertility – and even if they have – words can never do the experience any justice. It just doesn't happen. What will happen, though, are words being slung at you with great intentions that fall so short that you aren't even able to reach out and grab a couple for comfort. I found myself in many situations like this, which made me feel hurt, isolated, and even angry at other people who had no idea how their words made me feel. We must always give ourselves permission to feel the feelings and not let the inexperienced words of other people stick with us and take hold. Release them and move forwards. There are more critical things to do. You can't control what others say, but you can manage your process of dealing with these words. Journal out how you feel to help process their impact on how you think and move forward from them. Let these words flow over you.

We must be cautious of the expectations we place on people to speak the perfect words at the ideal time. When we share our experiences or challenges, we often don't want responses to pacify our discomfort. We want to be seen, felt, heard, and for people to understand our suffering. We're looking for connection and feeling cared for, for someone to sit in the emotional turmoil that we are in and hang out there with us.

Our human tendency is to try and make things better, often for our discomfort in someone else's pain. When people around us struggle, we try to help make the pain disappear. When the pain is chronic and not easily dismissed, it takes emotional intelligence and a level of vulnerability to stay present and acknowledge that words aren't going to help. The presence in pain is powerful. Even knowing and experiencing this, I gravitate towards "fixing" things for others to remove their pain and discomfort. It's not easy, so managing our expectations of others is helpful when navigating these situations.

Keep in focus people's *intentions*, rather than the actual words. Suppose we operate under the concept that everyone is doing the best they can and that the people we trust with personal information genuinely care about us. In that case, we can let go of the misplaced words that get blurted out in moments of people being human and feeling empathetic on our behalf. It's hard not to help, and it's hard to sit in the discomfort of someone else's pain. Giving ourselves space and others grace is the name of the game.

Infertility can take over our internal dialogue entirely if left unchecked. The sheer time and energy it takes to follow treatment plans and appointment schedules lend itself to taking over our headspace. Intentional tending to our minds comes in. You are so much more than your current fertility status, so keep your thoughts captive to live this truth out. When you notice yourself investing too much of your inner dialogue on the components of your fertility treatments that you can't control, or obsessing over every detail, work towards keeping these thoughts contained. Perhaps schedule a time in your day to "worry" as a strategy to manage these thoughts. Set a timer to journal your thoughts. Bring awareness to how much time and energy you want to allow your mind to take over, and assess where you are at with this. If this is an area of great struggle, connecting with a counselor to provide specific strategies may be an excellent option for you.

Certain situations can be ripe for overanalyzing. Family gatherings, baby showers, and birthday parties quickly become times of preemptive worry and anxiety about what others may say or how you may feel. When conversations focus entirely on babies and pregnancies, it will naturally stir up concern. Take some time to think through your plan or strategize before the party, arming yourself with potential responses that feel comfortable if a comment is made or an uncomfortable question may be asked. In this case, taking some time to be prepared can reduce the anxiety of being caught off guard. It allows the opportunity to speak the truth in a way that feels good and to limit the premature worry and stress about going to the event surrounding uncertainty. The conversations I'd come up with in my head often did not play out. This means some wasted worry, as much of what we worry about never comes to be. We can spend a specific length of time preparing for these situations, or we can drag on circular thought patterns, anticipating and worrying and draining ourselves. Having an anticipatory guard up interferes with enjoying events and time with people. Preparing responses can help you feel more comfortable entering high-pressure moments with a sense of control over your responses. Journaling your thoughts can help get them out on paper and reduce spiraling thought processes in your mind. Setting a time limit on journaling and preparations before an event can help limit the amount of energy you give to different situations. Mind your mind. Give grace to those asking and respond how you feel most comfortable.

Questions:

1. Scenario: You are at a baby shower for your best friend. Attending the event is a mix of friends and family members you don't know. You're sitting next to your friend's aunt, making conversation while the mother-to-be opens gifts. She asks you if you have any kids.
   1. What feelings do you think might come up for you?
   2. Brainstorm two possible ways you could respond in this situation.
2. Scenario: You are in a group of people discussing their children and the question of family planning and the number of desired children comes up.
   1. What feelings do you think might come up?
   2. Brainstorm two possible ways you could react to this situation.
3. What comments have people made to you that were hurtful? What do you think they were trying to communicate? How would you react differently if that situation were to happen again?
4. What are some phrases you can use to address unwanted comments? Some examples for when someone asks you when you are going to have children: "We are working hard on it," "We are hoping for the same thing," and "This is not a topic I'd like to discuss." Sometimes silence is best. Let the comment linger, and then carry on to a new topic.

5. Anticipating stressful events can often cause more stress than the event itself. Creating an action plan can help you feel prepared and reduce the stress of being caught off guard.

> 1. What specific situations are you most nervous about encountering? For example, someone asking if you plan to have kids? Being in an awkward position with others talking about their birth stories?
>
> 2. Create some of your own "If_(this happens)_, then_(I'll do this)_" strategies to help with the preparation and anticipatory processing.

BOUNDARIES TO PROTECT YOUR PARTNER RELATIONSHIP

Conversations about sperm count, embryo quality, or supporting a partner by administering injections likely weren't a part of your wedding vows or dialogue before family planning began. It's easy to find yourself and your partner's relationship totally thrown off through this time. Each partner navigates their unique experience and comes together to make decisions that may change the trajectory of their lives. All the while, you are trying to support one another in an exhausting season.

Open communication with your partner is critical. There are challenges when partners disagree on intervention boundaries when one person is ready to push forward, and the other may be digging in their heels for various reasons. This stirs up a lot of emotional turmoil, guilt, blame, and relational stress. Time can bring understanding, and viewing the situation from both sides is essential. It's important to empathize on behalf of one another as this level of stress can highlight the worst sides of ourselves. Where are they coming from? What is important for them? Counseling can be a great option to help process the conflicts as they arise when goals and ideas don't line up. Your relationship is valuable and worth the investment. The consequences of neglecting your relationship during this critical time can be disastrous. You chose each other first; remember that and invest in that.

Around the time we entered into our infertility journey, we had just become friends with a couple who were eight years ahead in their struggle. Experience nourishes wisdom. My friend told me to keep in mind that "you chose your husband first" – before the family we hope for, before the invasive treatments, before anything else. This was wise counsel at an opportune time, and a mindset that would help us maintain a healthy relationship through our upcoming challenges. She had seen too many people fixate on the process and outcome, neglecting the relationship that is the very essence and reason for the hope of children in the first place. I'm grateful for this wise counsel that set the tone for the years ahead.

It's easy when stretched and strained and emotionally empty to lose sight of the very reason you're fighting in the first place. Building a family with your partner requires a solid and sturdy foundation of a healthy relationship. I didn't always get this part right. It took bringing myself back to those words many times when feeling frustrated and burdened with the unevenly weighted part I played as a woman in the treatment process. It was easy for resentment to build, as most of the workload was on me based on biology alone.

Generally, it is more common for the workload to fall primarily on the female partner who hopes to carry the baby. However, this is not a universal experience. Depending on the nature of your relationship, it may be more heavily on your partner. It's necessary to keep in mind the mismatched workload that often exists, as this is an area that can provoke much resentment when left unchecked.

This unbalanced level of observable effort can be dramatic, leaving ample space for negative emotions and resentment to fester. There was a time when I was on a strict diet, eating my vegetables, lean meat, nuts and seeds and looking at Erik with rage as he ate his pizza and chips on a Friday night. Logically, I knew that my treatment plan involved following rigid guidelines to help improve egg quality. In contrast, Erik's plan was much less intensive, requiring a few supplements to maintain his health. I understood the science, but I didn't like its reality. It started to fester and get to me. When I finally shared with him that it made me frustrated to see him living his everyday life when mine had to be altered in every way imaginable, he heard me, and it made sense to him. Altering how I spent my time, changes to my work, adjustments to my diet, shifts in my hormones, all of these changes to follow my plan. It was helpful for him to hear it from my perspective, which brought clarity to the frustration and anger I was subconsciously expressing towards him without even realizing it. After talking it through, he agreed he would track with me on the dietary changes so that I wasn't alone in this area.

In those moments of frustration, I failed to realize the emotional burden he was quietly carrying for the both of us. He took the weight of my challenges while staying strong and optimistic that things would work out okay. The burden is still very present on the partner not preparing to carry a child. It is challenging on both ends, and since partners who aren't carrying a child can't change the fact that they don't typically play a prominent role in the process, it's not fair to hold it against them. Open communication and sharing small areas of frustration as they come up will help to dissipate the massive eruptions of bottled-up emotions.

Look for the gestures of compassion and understanding, and ask for what you need. Without sharing specific needs, we can't expect these needs to be met. The emotions surrounding uncertainty are felt equally by each partner. Even though your partner may not be experiencing everything that you are, your home *is*. Bring acute awareness of what you need and learn to ask for it. If you don't have clarity on what you need, your partner will most certainly be in the dark about it. Asking your partner about their needs can help build understanding and support for your relationship during this season. Infertility has the potential to make or break relationships. Establishing reliable communication can help set you up for success while going through treatment and beyond.

How do we have boundaries with our internal dialogue about our partners? When resentment, anger, and hurt set in, and the narrative in our head creates an enemy-ship in our relationship, how do we stop the runaway mental chatter that seeks to pull us apart on the journey? Rein in your thoughts. Remember that you are in this together, not battling against one another. Resentment is poison in a relationship. John Gottman and Nan Silver's *The Seven*

Principles for Making Marriage Work[19] is an excellent resource for fostering successful relationships. Concepts include pulling away from the conflict at hand and honoring your relationship even when your partner doesn't do it right. Emotional fragility, uncharted relationship territory, and exhaustion make relationships incredibly hard. Suit up and commit to prioritizing you and your partner's needs as you work as a team to build your family.

Find Ways to Keep Things Light

Life is heavy during this time, and can quickly feel like you are carrying an extra 100 pounds. In times of heaviness, it takes work to have moments where things are light. Find little ways to release pressure along the way to avoid a build-up of emotions that becomes too much to manage and contain. Laughter is the universal language of keeping things light. A gentle release, even a little bit, is helpful when emotions start to build. Don't lose this – don't give away your laughter. The infertility process can threaten it on a good day, yet being diligent and aware can help keep things light.

We drove down to the city, all geared up with anxious anticipation of our first egg retrieval for our IVF. We made a point of "making a day of it." Rather than driving a few hours for one appointment, we would attach a meal or shopping trip around the event to spread our focus and inject some fun into the mix. The retrieval went smoothly overall, and I felt terrific after a short nap post-procedure. The medication concoction was on the strong side, so I didn't feel any level of pain. We took our post-op instruction sheet the nurse handed to us along with our hopeful aspirations. We were on our way out of the clinic, carrying on with our day of fun.

We had gift certificates to The Keg and Cineplex we had saved for this special occasion. We took the opportunity to commemorate our procedure day with a tasty dinner and a movie date. The steak, potatoes, and salad had never tasted so good. After dinner, we opted for a light-hearted movie, *Zootopia*, to cap off the day before heading home. I had been a little more tired than anticipated – in fact; I was absentminded from the drugs I'd been given for my procedure – which I didn't realize until after the movie. Following the plot was challenging, and I was fighting off sleep the entire time. A few weeks later, a TV commercial for *Zootopia* came on, and I asked Erik if we had seen that movie. We just laughed as we put the pieces of that day together. This will always be a funny memory for us. Perhaps enjoying a chill time at home may be more applicable to keep things light while following post-op instructions.

As we prepared for our second IVF egg retrieval, we decided to stay the night before in a hotel to reduce travel stress and enjoy our time *before* the procedure, unlike our mistake from our previous adventure. We settled into our hotel room and enjoyed some time relaxing, eating good food, and watching light-hearted TV before resting up.

The following day, we walked to the appointment from our hotel, understanding what was ahead since we had been there before. We were prepped and ready to go, waiting and all gowned up for the procedure. I looked at Erik and had a good chuckle at the image of him wearing his scrubs. He is needle-phobic and practically all medical procedure-phobic, so it was a funny sight at that moment. Anxiety mixed with camaraderie and unity of us in this experience together had us laughing at each other in our medical gear. Keeping things light helped one of our heaviest moments become a pleasant memory.

These were pivotal moments in time. Certain times can easily be overcome with the intensity of our emotions that we lose out on the moment if we aren't careful. While our anxieties can have us fully in the future of what-ifs, there's true beauty in *living* these moments in all of their complexity. They weren't wholly joyful, yet there was joy infused in the complexity of it all. We carried this same concept of keeping things light as we started working through our adoption application. In the stress of these times, we can easily get caught up in the *doing* and less in the *being*. Keeping things light and finding laughter along the way is helpful.

We completed our dossier and our adoption paperwork package. It was ready to be mailed on a beautiful warm, windy day. These papers were the final pieces of a massive puzzle, representing the grueling process we'd been through. We had endured months of paperwork, police fingerprinting, background checks, medicals, psychological assessments, parenting courses, and home study evaluations. It was a monumental day for the future direction of our family. We were mailing these finalized documents and photos to our agency before going out for a celebratory dinner at a local Thai food restaurant. We walked together to the mailbox just outside our nearby drug store. Erik was placing the mail in the slot when the wind snatched it out of his hands, causing it to blow away along the pavement. I kid you not. I chased it for about ten steps before taking hold and firmly placed it in the slot to be mailed off. "That's it. It's never going to happen for us!" We both laughed. We loved the irony and visual that the final piece of the adoption process in our control was blown away by the wind. Keep things light and keep laughing.

Infertility can cause our blessings to be in our blind spots. Regularly recount blessings and intentionally seek out joy during difficult times.

FINAL THOUGHTS

SUPPORTING PEOPLE
THROUGH INFERTILITY

Mother's Day has been difficult since my mom passed away in 2009.

Having experienced a miscarriage and several years of fertility treatments, the pain of this day is naturally compounded. Everything stings and seems to be felt more deeply on days like this. Days meant to highlight and celebrate the sacrificial love of mothers.

We attend church most Sunday mornings, but through the years, I learned that it was best to skip church on Mother's Day. This strategy helped avoid the inevitable tear fest in public, which is not my idea of a fun time. One year, I felt optimistic and decided to attend church on a particular Mother's Day. It was a charming service, and I was managing well. Very smoothly, in fact, until the last five minutes.

Our pastor gave special acknowledgment to people who are suffering. He spoke to those who have lost a child, those unable to have children, and those who have lost or have a difficult relationship with their mother: check, check, check. I completely lost it, and my poised and contained demeanor was shaken.

I mean no blame to our pastor. To have a service and speak only of the joys of motherhood when there is real suffering and sorrow would be a disservice to so many. It was the straw that broke the camel's back for me. The service held *hundreds* of people, and we were sitting towards the front. It wasn't a cute little tear that I dabbed off with a tissue. It was a full-on ugly cry, and I had to leave the church to contain myself. It would have been entirely disruptive for me to stay, and it was disruptive to go.

From then on, I decided to remove myself from the triggering situation and enjoy time to do whatever I needed to do on Mother's Day. Our needs can change every year, that's okay. Flexibility and checking in with ourselves are vital. Some years I celebrate with my step-mom and mother-in-law, and other years I don't. Honoring your needs involves removing judgment from your decisions. It's simple, and yet it can have a profound impact.

Recipe for managing Mother's Day (or any other challenging day):

- **Remain schedule-free.** By keeping your day free of plans, you leave it open to whatever feels best for that day. Sometimes you may feel great and want to invest your time in a way that honors feeling great, whatever that is for you. Sometimes sadness may feel overwhelming, which is normal and okay. In this case, you will appreciate that you don't have to cancel plans or feel the need to "push through" at a function you aren't feeling up to. Sometimes you will feel like any other day and look forward to spending quality time with family honoring your mother or a mother-figure in your life. I'm currently writing this on Mother's Day, and so far today, I have enjoyed sleeping in, baking, tidying up, going for a long run, having a bath, and lounging around. It has been the perfect day.

- **Avoid social media.** Don't peek, don't scroll. At all. Just don't. You don't need additional cues to prompt jealousy, anger, frustration, sadness, or pain. The feelings are there, and they don't need to be exacerbated or convoluted by other people displaying their joy of motherhood or people singing praises of the mothers in their lives. It's too much, and it moves us too quickly into a comparison mindset triggering deep grief, which we know is not helpful. Stay in your lane here and tune in to how you feel separate from other people's experiences.

- **Be gentle with yourself.** It's okay to have many feelings, and it's okay to have none at all. Today we had the Blue Jays game on in the background, and the announcer commented that one of the players was celebrating his first Mother's Day without his mom. She had passed away not long before. He had a great hit, and they mentioned that he was playing for his mom. That did it for me. I cried. Letting it out is part of this process. Remind yourself that no feeling is a bad feeling. Express what you need to when you need to express it. It's all a healthy part of grief. Do a little, feel a little.

- **Create a plan to celebrate your mother.** If you have a mother or mother figure that you are celebrating, there are many ways that you can do this while leaving space for yourself to grieve. You can give flowers, baked goods, or a letter of gratitude, to name a few. These can be delivered ahead of time if you need space, or shared on the day may be a nice distraction as you engage in showing love to the remarkable women in your life.

For Those Supporting Someone Going Through Infertility

The journey of infertility is meant to be shouldered and shared. As painful of an experience as infertility is, supporting someone going through it can be very painful. Feelings of helplessness can be provoked by not knowing what to say, how to help, or what to do while someone you love is suffering. It's okay not to know. Offering support often looks very different depending on everyone's individual needs and the day. Here are some helpful hints from someone who has received various levels of support and what I found to be helpful:

- Ask. A kind thing to do is ask what support is needed. Ask if it's helpful to let them know that you are thinking about them. Ask if they want you to ask about their treatments or wait for them to bring it up to protect their privacy. Ask if there is a better way to support them right now.

- Offer advice only if you are explicitly asked for advice. Listening is therapy. So often, the problems, uncertainty, and stress of the situation just need to be verbalized to someone who is actively listening and able to empathize. Listening with a compassionate ear is validating and so appreciated.

- Your presence matters. You may feel like you aren't doing enough because you aren't "doing" anything to help the situation. Being available and being present is more meaningful than you think.

- Research. Learn about the procedures your loved one goes through to understand what is going on. This is an act of love. If they have to explain the medical procedures, it can take away from the emotions and stress of the situation, which is the more critical area of support that is needed.

- Support their decisions. It can be hard to watch someone continue something that is causing so much pain, and it's hard to understand why anyone would subject themselves to something so intense and challenging. Respect their desire to build their family and acknowledge their strength and courage to pursue treatments. Acknowledge their strength and courage to stop or choose not to pursue treatments.

- Remember them on Mother's Day and Father's Day. These are challenging days. A gentle note or delivery of flowers or another small gesture are thoughtful ways to let them know they aren't forgotten.

Things to avoid saying when someone is going through infertility:

- Relax. It's not helpful, and it's nearly impossible to do. Highlighting the stress is painful and invalidating.

- Minimizing the problem. Saying things like "enjoy your time as the two of you," "enjoy your sleep while you can get it," and "at least you can travel" are painful. Comments like these minimize a brutal journey.

- Offer solutions. Don't suggest they look into fertility treatments or adoption. Someone's family-building process needs to be processed and worked through. It's not a quick decision, and it's not for anyone else to decide but themselves.

- At least: "at least you have one child," "at least you are healthy." This minimizes the pain and is not kind or empathetic, highlighting that you don't understand. It feels like a shaming comment.

- Don't gossip. If someone has shared their infertility with you, private and personal information is meant to stay with you. Having anyone else circle back and discuss this information is intrusive and a massive break in trust.

- Don't pry for information. Allow someone to share the details they are comfortable sharing. Asking if it's someone's "fault" is too personal and can feel like blame is placed somewhere.

- Complain about your pregnancy. If you are pregnant and friends with someone infertile, they are not the person to complain to about your pregnancy symptoms. It's hard enough to be around pregnant people, and having them complain about what they are desperate to experience can be hard.

It's tough to support someone along this journey that can last many years. Having boundaries to ensure that you are offering support and not taking their burdens on for yourself is crucial for sustaining this type of support. You are a valuable part of your loved one's journey. Their thanks will be felt when they are on the other end of the battle when they can see how critical of a role you played. Thank you, on behalf of them right now, for being necessary support.

ACKNOWLEDGING AND PREVENTING BURNOUT

Burnout is a condition that I see in the office often. People come to see me after a period of extreme, sustained stress, then feel utterly awful on the other end of it. Without understanding the context of how they feel, they expect to feel much better once the stressor is removed or the time has passed, and things feel less urgent. Our catecholamines, stress hormones, compensate for the additional stressors. We aren't meant to live in a sustained experience of stress for a long time. The consequences during or after the stressful time can impact both mental and physical health. In this section, I refer to my own experience with burnout, treating burnout in my work, and the work of Amelia Nakoski and Emily Nagoski in their book, *Burnout: The Secret to Unlocking the Stress Cycle*[18].

Nagoski[18] discusses the importance of turning towards your own body with kindness and compassion, taking a break from things that cause stress and dealing with stress's impact on you. The concept is that stress is a cycle that you work through to release to prevent it from getting "stuck" and layered, inevitably leading to burnout. We work to release this stress and complete the cycles by physical activity to help your body process the stress, imagination such as daydreaming or reading a book or watching a movie, creative self-expression, or connection (with people, nature, animals, spirituality).

Starting IVF felt like a gun going off at the start of a race. The finish line, for me, was burnout. The very structure of infertility treatments lends itself to over-functioning on all levels, emotional, physical, mental, and spiritual. I wish I knew then what I know now. If I had known how stressful it was at the time, if I had turned to my body with kindness and compassion, I would have been able to move through it in a much healthier way.

I was ready for our final round of IVF to be over before we even began. I had just enough reserves to complete this last cycle in my heart, but my spirit was weak. In the eight months leading up to it, I expended my energy following a rigorous egg quality optimization protocol of clean eating and taking about 25 different supplements daily of specific herbs and nutraceuticals. All of this before starting the medications required for the medical procedure itself. My treatment plan included weekly Traditional Chinese Medicine (TCM) acupuncture sessions for 12 weeks. The acupuncturist was a former medical doctor from China. She would look at my tongue and eyes and check my pulses to evaluate how my body was doing and what needed attention that day. She told me on my first visit that I was exhausted, to which I corrected her and let her know that I was very energetic and enjoyed a very active and busy lifestyle. "I'm a high-capacity person who accomplishes a lot in a day. I'm not tired at all. In fact, I have loads of energy," I would say. After our first session, I went home and napped for three hours – I completely crashed. The following week, she said that I was drained and needed more rest. Resting was difficult during this season. I was energized by fear and fueled by adrenaline while not acknowledging the complete emotional and physical exhaustion I felt.

The winter after our treatments were done, I was sick four times. This was unusual for me. That winter was evidence of the strain my body had endured. It had been carrying a heavy burden for so long that I didn't feel it until it was lifted. The recovery from infertility-induced burnout took time as my body and mind caught up to the overtly physical and emotional strain. Recovery was rocky, requiring several days of "crashing" and laying in bed on the weekends. Patches of eczema showed up on my face, which I had never experienced before, and my hair started falling out at an increased rate. My body had been bending and adapting to stress, and it broke down when it didn't have to hang on any longer. The body levels up to challenges when facing stressors.

Amazingly, we can rev up stress hormones that give us superhuman energy and drive us through the stressor. We simply aren't meant to live there for extended periods. People are often diagnosed with PTSD in the infertility world, regardless of the outcome of the experience. It is traumatic, overwhelming, and grueling. Treat yourself with gentleness, compassion, and kindness if you are deep in it. Your body, mind and soul need it. Take breaks to come up for air. Pace yourself. Take steps every day to address and work through your stress while meeting the additional demands on your body.

Being outside of stress provides a new perspective. The process of learning to listen to your body evolves over time. Amid stress, it is essential to give ourselves permission to pause and plug into things that bring joy and promote relaxation. Checking in with our bodies and listening to how it feels and what needs tending to can be a healthy practice. Rest is required to keep going. This fight is draining. Infertility cuts a big hole in your cup, requiring regular re-fills to avoid completely emptying yourself. Personal needs are higher during this time.

Identifying warning signs that your body is being overworked or is under stress provide valuable insight during the experience of infertility and beyond. It takes time to learn what these early alarm bells are for you. An article in Forbes Magazine, *10 Signs You're Burning Out*, identifies exhaustion, cynicism and negative emotions, lack of motivation, cognitive concerns or difficulty focusing, reduced productivity and performance, increased conflicts with others or withdrawing from relationships, reduced self-care, becoming preoccupied with work (or fertility treatments), feeling dissatisfied, health concerns (like digestive issues, weight gain, depression)[13]. Prioritizing self-care prevents burnout and offers more significant levels of energy, improved mood, and increased resilience to life's challenges as they come up.

Exhaustion can be a scary place. It can make you feel like a shell of who you know you are. It is not a place we are meant to camp out for long periods. Consider the discomfort of this exhaustion to be a self-check point. It's startling enough to force change, which the body desperately communicates. It's a warning sign. Life can't keep going like this. It is a time to evaluate what is critically important and must remain and tune in to what needs to be shed to build back a more resilient version of you.

Rest and self-care look different for each of us. For myself, it includes moving my body, having meaningful conversations, spending quality time with my family, eating well, and occasionally scheduling a weekend without any plans. Watching things grow and observing changes in nature as the seasons change is an enjoyable, peaceful way to incorporate mindfulness into my life. Discovering something that makes me happy and trying new things has been a healing part of my journey to finding myself again.

A few months ago, we were hiking Angel's Landing at Zion National Park. It's a steep climb with a particularly challenging switchback section. It was hot and grueling. We traded off carrying our backpack throughout the climb that contained our water and food. It happened to be my turn to take the pack during the start of this steep section. Partway through, I offloaded the backpack to Erik and was reminded that we don't know how heavy a load is until it's gone. We adapt and adjust when heavy is the norm and life keeps happening. Life can feel heavy when we don't realize it, and we don't feel the load while carrying it. We can only manage so much emotional weight until we reach capacity. My emotional baggage was interfering with my ability to cope with day-to-day challenges, and I didn't realize it until it was over.

Healing happens in time. Different seasons in life hold different purposes and capacities. Limit energy exertion outside of your immediate needs. The demand internally is more significant than we can see or fully know while currently in it. Focus on completing stress cycles regularly by implementing systematic strategies while managing the heavy load of infertility.

Practical Strategies to Prevent Burnout:

Stay connected to the things that make you feel alive, energized, and spark joy. The things that make you, *you*. Take time to reflect on your changing needs as you navigate your journey. What makes you, *you*? Are you a social person who requires quality time with friends and family? Don't lose sight of that. Prioritize it. Are you someone who recharges on your own? Schedule downtime to re-energize. It's an exhausting process that requires a lot of interaction, which can be draining. Do you enjoy being connected in your community? Plug into a community group that allows you to give back and use your strengths. Involving yourself in meaningful work outside of yourself is a great way to change your focus. Whatever it looks like for you, spend time thinking this through to ensure that you aren't losing sight of the things that make you who you are.

Burnout is becoming an increasingly common experience. Over time, chronic stress and overworking wear the body and soul down, and it happens inside and outside of infertility battles. Specific measures can help support your body's additional load as you navigate this season.

- **Move your body.** This is the top strategy for managing

stress and improving well-being. It helps to enhance the brain's sensitivity to serotonin (our "happy hormone"), boosts endorphins and self-confidence. Move in a way that you enjoy. Trail walking/running, swimming, biking, fitness classes, or yoga to help calm the nervous system. Personally, I enjoy exercising outdoors with friends. Listen to your body and do what works for you.

- **Connection.** We are designed to connect with others, and our brain and body are designed for this, introverts and extroverts alike. Spending time with people we love builds us up and helps us feel safe. Hugging releases oxytocin and offers emotional release, and supports our physical bodies going through so much through these treatments. Connecting with pets, nature, or a higher power has been shown to have the same positive response to relieving stress. Find your sense of connection.

- **Rest.** Create a routine and rhythm that incorporates rest each day. Tend to your emotional health and incorporate solitude and self-reflection. Rest is critical for preventing burnout, and you need more rest than you will likely feel comfortable giving yourself. In this focus on rest, quality sleep is vital as well. It's when our brain and body *genuinely* rest. Carve out downtime in the evening to wind down from the day to maximize quality sleep at night.

- **Play.** Life is heavy when dealing with a potential loss of hopes and dreams with the uncertainty of building your family. Emotions are all-consuming, and plans are weaving in and out of reality. Spending time being creative or doing things for fun can help shift the mind from the task lists and stress mode to rest. Creative self-expression in any form is a way to release stress from the body. What did you enjoy doing as a child? If you love arts and crafts, grab a coloring book or start an art project to connect with your creative side. Following strict guidelines and regimes can be draining. Balance your brain with creative outlets to give your mind a break.

- **Journal.** Take some time to put your thoughts and feelings on paper. This is a great way to help process your emotions, bring clarity to your thoughts, and help organize the complexity of the process. Things can get confusing, layered, and muddled easily. Write it out, sit with it, and work through what's coming up for you along the way.

- **Cry.** Let yourself feel your feelings and release them. Crying releases cortisol and adrenaline, which helps balance your emotions, rather than building up in your body.

- **Healthy Fuel.** You don't burn out from eating poorly, but it does impact how you feel. Fueling our body with healthy food allows the proper fuel to provide consistent energy and the building blocks needed for our bodies to function optimally. The demands on the body are much higher during treatments, and stress can influence the food choices we make. Feed your body healthy food at least 80 percent of the time to give your body the basic requirements for your health. Focusing on a healthy whole foods diet supports fertility efforts and prevents the negative consequences of a diet high in processed foods (lower mood, sluggish feeling, fatigue). Eating well helps us feel well. Focus on eating whole foods. Fuel your body for function.

Tips for healthy eating:

- Eat a protein source with each meal (meat, fish, beans, legumes, nuts, seeds, eggs, etc.).

- Eat various vegetables and fruit (nutrient-dense foods high in fiber help you feel full).

- Eat whole grains in place of refined grains (oats, quinoa, brown rice, whole grains).

- Hydrate primarily with water (aim for nearly clear urine).

- Limit sugar, caffeine, processed foods and alcohol (which can impact energy, mood, and stress).

- 80:20 Rule (eat healthy foods 80% of the time and remain

flexible for social gatherings and engage in food for enjoyment).

Stress and worry don't change an outcome; however, they drain our resources. Stress is constant during infertility, and it adds weight to an already heavy load. It is a beneficial, clarifying practice to consciously separate in our minds what *can* be controlled (taking medications, getting to the appointments, having bloodwork done) from the things that *can't* (outcome, timeline, knowing what the next steps will be). Focusing on the actionable steps, rather than the theoretical possibilities, helps us invest our precious energy and reduce unnecessary drain. Physical and mental energy are limited; aim to minimize the waste of precious resources on things that can't be controlled. Thinking harder or analyzing longer doesn't change the outcome. Life's load is heavy. Make sure that what you are carrying is critical in helping you to move forward, not weighing you down. Acknowledge that this season is stressful, and the needs your body and mind have due to the increase in stress are high and valid. Implement strategies that address and meet these needs.

Questions:

1. What are your body's warning signs that you are stressed?
2. Brainstorm activities that are restful for you.
3. When was the last time you gave yourself permission to rest? How did that feel?

4. Carve out time each day to listen to what your body needs. Be specific in making a time to do this.
5. What does your current life load feel like? Heavy? Light? Overwhelming? Balanced?
6. What causes you to feel heavy and weighed down?
7. What burnout prevention strategies do you want to focus on?

MY FAITH AND INFERTILITY

———⁓⁓———

For the past few years, I have highlighted a "word of the year" for the year ahead. It's a way to place an overarching focus for the year and work towards something meaningful. I find it to be an excellent alternative to New Year's resolutions that can often be shaming and surface-level changes we hope to achieve that fall flat within days or weeks. It's been neat to look back on these words and how they have served me and encapsulated these past few years.

Word of the Year: Surrender

In 2017, I chose "surrender" as my word for the year during treatments. We would be completing our second and final IVF, and I would ultimately need to surrender to whatever this year brought our way. My intention to surrender the process and outcome allowed me to release the desire of clinging too tightly to an outcome that could not be controlled. The harsh reality of infertility is that we can control getting to our appointments, taking medications as directed and following instructions from our health care team, the outcome remains harshly outside our control. My life and these plans are not my own. Why remain in a struggle against the ultimate direction we are meant to go? When I fully embraced this experience of surrendering and letting go, I could let myself "be" and trust in the greater perspective and purpose.

The rhythm of music has always been more engaging than the lyrics themselves, and it's what catches my attention first. As I've grown, the lyrics of a song have become more meaningful as music relates to my life experiences. I can listen to a song several times without paying attention to the meaning of the words. Through life's challenges of the last decade of my life, music became much more about lyrics and connecting through shared experiences. It's become therapeutic and purposeful.

While traveling to one of my routine ultrasound monitoring appointments near the start of my treatments, a new song on the radio station caught my attention. The first time I heard this song, it brought me to tears. It felt so pointed with the overwhelming disappointment of that season. The lyrics of "Trust in You" by Lauren Daigle started, "Letting go of every single dream, I lay each one down at your feet".[14] Laying down my dreams was not my initial reaction and didn't feel natural. I wanted to fight for these dreams. Fighting for the outcome to be within *my* control, I would simply work harder, do more, test further, treat more. Laying down my family dreams at the feet of God has required conviction and has been the most challenging spiritual experience in my life to date. Relinquishing control was unnatural and completely necessary. This act of intentional surrender was freeing, and this song highlighted and supported this process for me during this time.

I can vividly remember a conversation with a good friend shortly after my miscarriage several years ago, before any treatments had begun. I told her about my fear of how long it might take us to get pregnant again, knowing it was more than an eight-year journey for other close friends. That was unfathomable at the time. In the back of my mind, I felt that this friendship might be a foreshadowing or preparation for the struggle ahead of us. This wasn't a struggle I wanted to face. My friend told me to pray about it – pray that it wouldn't take that long and that the journey would be over soon. I couldn't. At that time, I could not surrender that part of my life. The desire to have control was so strong that surrendering wasn't something I felt I could do. As though this would somehow prevent the struggle. It seems silly now that I thought I had any control over this. There was an ignorance there that highlighted a character weakness needing attention.

Over the next several months, this song would consistently play on the radio on the way to appointments, and it became my steady reminder to let go of this need to control. As challenging as these words were to listen to and truly live out, it was this process of surrender and letting go that I needed so desperately. I *was* weary, needed emotional rest, and needed to trust in the One who holds my life in His hands. Trusting and letting go is unnatural for me. For many of us, it seems. We want to predict our future, plan and prepare for it, know what to expect and when. Whether you believe in God or a higher power, an acknowledgment is required that our human experience doesn't offer us endless control of outcomes. We want it to, we think we can, but we can't. Surrendering is an active process in releasing outcomes and trusting in something greater than ourselves.

Many of our typical responses to challenges are approaching them head-on. We don't want to wait and see how things play out. Committing, making a plan, and making things happen feels more manageable. This has been a refining process for me. Letting go and letting God take the reins has been humbling and anxiety-relieving. Trusting and surrendering in this process has not been easy. The lyrics of this song spoke to me when I needed them the most. We always want our hopes, dreams, and prayers to lead to the outcome we think is best. I've learned that what I think is best is not always what God has in store, and His plans are perfect. Trusting in God and His plans has brought peace through this experience. Allowing life to unfold in a different, even more fantastic way. It has allowed me to see that whatever the outcome, whatever the timeline, the One who made the stars and the mountains and vast oceans, holds my present and my future, which is good and for good.

The further we embarked on the medical treatments, the tighter I clung to the outcomes. I picture a child who will not sleep when their parents get them ready for bed. They keep getting out of bed, crying, whining, becoming inconsolable. The best thing for them is to stop resisting, yet their persistence to stay up longer gets stronger and stronger as time goes on. Eventually, their body gives in and accepts that it needs rest, and all is well and peaceful in the home again. The greater the fight, the harder it is for everyone involved and the more emotionally taxing and more challenging it is to reason within the moment.

Without fail, this song would play on route to essential appointments, on days of our IUIs. We were driving to an IVF appointment in silence, and when I turned on the radio, this song was playing. More recently, we were in the process of buying a home outside of the city, one we had hoped to raise our son in. The night we were meeting to negotiate the deal, it came on the radio after a few years without hearing it. The message came through loud and clear. When we remain open to learning and growing through challenging experiences, we keep open to many important lessons. We went on to buy the house, and I was able to surrender that decision while listening to the lyrics in our car before the deal came to a close.

Word of the Year: Adventure

In 2018, we completed our fertility treatments, which offered the freedom to engage in life again in a new way. It was a much-needed break and an opportunity to shift gears, gain perspective, and redirect energy. My word for this year was "adventure," as I had worked on surrendering our family plan and was ready to see our change in direction and life moving forward as an adventure. It was a helpful way to lighten up the heaviness of life for the past few years.

Heading home for lunch one day, an upbeat song on the radio caught my attention (I remember the volume being low, but I was feeling the happy beat). Turning up the volume revealed a fun, lighthearted, happy song. I was gravitating towards this type of light music after what had been a heavy season.

Matthew Parker's song, *Adventure, contained* lyrics that were exactly what I needed to hear. "Life is black and blue, happy then it's sad, just call it an *adventure,* then it ain't so bad."[15] It was such a friendly reminder and quite literally encapsulated the sentiments of my word for the year. This word and song helped to shift my mindset. Being ready to move forward and reframe my thinking as we transitioned into this new stage of our journey allowed this song to be a fun reminder of this change of season. We were on such a wild roller coaster ride, and it was an adventure. Though the challenges of our journey were far from over, reframing this season from feeling the fear of the unknown to seeing it as an adventure had been an intentional, positive shift.

Adventure is defined as "an exciting or remarkable experience... an undertaking usually involving danger and unknown risks."[16] Our family-building journey fits this definition. Though the hardships and losses of this journey are not one that we would have chosen, the experience in its entirety and the outcome have been quite the adventure, worth every moment. Our understanding of building a family has certainly involved a level of boldness and risk, and our future is exciting and full of adventure. Traveling to Thailand to meet and bring our son home during the COVID-19 pandemic, it doesn't get more adventurous than that! This new word of focus helped us view obstacles through our adoption journey as character-building opportunities. There is way less stress involved when thinking and problem-solving from this mindset. It also helped in our pursuit of keeping things light.

It's amazing for music to speak into different seasons of life. It can be powerful and transformative and remind us that we aren't alone in our situations or journeys. I love the line in this song that says, "Our dreams will come alive."[15] They will, and they are. For you, too.

Word of the Year: Savor

Fast forward to the present day, 2021. We are home with our son Pete and settling into our groove as new parents to a unique, energetic toddler. These past years have been a whirlwind of effortful forward motion that has been starkly contrasted with slowing down and savoring where we are now. It's a sweet season of learning all about Pete: who he is, his likes and dislikes, what brings him joy, what causes him fear. Days, weeks, and months simply continue to go by. The purposeful steps of the past several years are replaced with intentional actions of our current reality in parenting. Having Pete doesn't cause the time to stand still, though I wish it would sometimes. Still, my mind is engaged in thinking of what may be to come for Pete and our family. The dreams, the struggles, the hardships, and the celebrations. Our natural tendency to imagine and anticipate our futures don't stop once a child enters our home.

I am savoring it. Savoring this precious child in our family and savoring his toddler antics and silly ways. Savoring his songs and dances. Savoring the "mommy up's" and the "I love you's." I am savoring the precious kisses and bedtime snuggles.

The transition from wishing life could be lived in fast forward to having the family we have been waiting for reminds us to savor the present moment. Life is valuable in every season. There is a purpose for each season. No season is best lived in fast forward. No season is wasted. There is an opportunity to savor along the way. There will never be the available time for you or you as a couple as before children. You will never get that back. There will never be more available mental capacity to process your thoughts and reflect on life. Do your best to savor it. We can't rewind time.

This forward motion is persistent, relentless. In our few months at home, Pete has gained a couple of pounds, grown an inch, and is growing up before our very eyes. So we do our best to savor it. To slow down and take in the moments that life offers us. The good, the bad, the happy, the sad. All of it.

My challenge is this: be present where you are and soak it all in. You can experience conflicting emotions at the same time. You can feel the intense frustration and sadness of infertility while savoring quality time with yourself or your partner. You can be devastated by the losses of infertility and savor the hope of what your family will come to be. Feel both. Let yourself feel both.

Questions:

1. As triggering situations come up, ask yourself if this will matter in five days, five months, or five years from now, and use it as a tool for gaining perspective.
2. Choose a word for your year. How do you want to see it shape the year ahead?
3. How can you harness the power of savoring your current

circumstances?

4. What will you look forward to savoring in the next stage of your journey?

SEASONS CHANGE

―⁓⁓―

Winter in Ontario can be pretty brutal. They're long and dreary, the kind of season that requires a deep breath at the start to gear up for what's ahead. An intentional action plan will help you savor it and enjoy the beauty while navigating the challenges that come with it. Just as winter comes in with all of the weight it can carry and all the challenges it brings, spring is sure to follow. Temperatures start to rise, the ground softens, and beautiful plants that were dormant for a time begin to emerge. Seasons change.

Spring has come to our corner of the world. I am writing this final chapter on a balcony in Bangkok, Thailand, less than two days away from meeting our son. Our adoption journey had been pretty smooth, and the paperwork was meticulous, but we made our way through it, eager to move forward and meet our son.

In the winter of 2020, we went on a holiday to San Diego to enjoy a mini winter escape and quality time together as a couple. We enjoyed a relaxed morning. On the first day of our trip didn't have a plan or schedule. The phone rang. A phone call that I will never forget: "I am calling to let you know that you are a mom!" I sobbed happy tears that day, more than I ever have in my entire life. I'm brought to tears any time I think of this phone call. We were matched with our son Pete that day, an unimaginably exciting time. We sat together and savored the moment; a moment cemented in our memory bank. We saw photos of our son for the first time that day, and our lives would never be the same again.

We arrived home from San Diego 13 days before the COVID-19 pandemic became a conversation in our province, and restrictions started being enforced. We will all remember where we were at this time in history and the personal impact it would bring. For us, it brought much uncertainty around our adoption and meeting our son.

Life doesn't quit. When facing challenges, we hope that surviving each one will protect us from the next hit, a time where we can insulate ourselves from hardship. One challenge helps to build resiliency and prepares us for the next. Undoubtedly, life is full of challenges. Our season of uncertainty with infertility helped prepare us for the delay that COVID-19 brought to our family. We didn't know how our travel to Thailand would be affected, but we had faced uncertainty before. The original plan was to travel to Thailand to meet our son in October 2020, eight months from when we were matched with him. We had no information about when our trip would take place until November 2020. It was unsettling to live with so many weighty unknowns while grieving our separation from our son. Uncertainty, in this case, was like a muscle that we had been working out. Unfamiliar situations allow us to adapt and change our thinking to make the experience smoother.

We channeled our energy towards preparing and mailing a care package to Thailand a few months after being matched with Pete. It was a specific combination of items for him to enjoy while we waited for the go-ahead to travel and bring him home. Included in the package was a photo album with English/Thai phrases for him to get to know us and become familiar with our faces. We also sent a book with our recorded voices reading a children's story, a teddy bear from our trip to San Diego where we first learned he was our son, a blanket that lived in our bed for a few weeks to absorb our smell, and a Toronto Raptors ball, to welcome the newest fan member to the club. It was an area where we could take action, which felt purposeful, and we started bonding with our son on the other side of the world.

We spent time organizing, purging, and cleaning our home during our wait and increased time at home with the lockdowns in place. Nesting began. We painted and prepared Pete's room to get everything ready for when we got the go-ahead to travel. In early fall 2020, an opportunity came up to move to a farmhouse outside the city. We looked over the previous year for homes that offered more space to raise our son. We fell in love with the house and decided to move in the middle of a pandemic, even though we didn't know when we would be traveling to Thailand. We moved 12 days before flying to Bangkok while continuing to work full-time. We will never forget this time in our lives! We were thankful we had invested energy in the purging of our home ahead of time at the start of the pandemic – not a minute was spared from that point forward.

We make plans, review them, share them, change them, and

the reality is that these revised plans ultimately change *us*. We know we never have control in the first place. The perfectly put-together bedroom, painted with the perfect color of green/blue/grey, wasn't the bedroom for Pete. We don't always know what the future holds. Trust in the process and direction rather than fixating on outcomes. It may be better than you can imagine, and it certainly has been for us. We have gained absolute beauty from ashes.

My three sisters hosted an adoption shower for me on a beautiful summer day. On the drive to the shower, I was filled with emotions. I welcomed the feelings, allowing myself to acknowledge what I was feeling, and the complexities of it all. The uncertainty of our travel schedule. The gratitude for what we were celebrating. The pain of having a son in a different country. The joy of being surrounded by close friends and family. I let myself feel the feelings, of which there were many that day.

Beautiful music came from outdoor speakers and a stunning garden party surrounded by mature trees in my stepmom's backyard. There were bright floral tablecloths, beautiful flower arrangements on the tables, a children's book for the guest book, and succulents as party gifts for the guests that my sister had been propagating for months. We enjoyed an incredible spread of my favorite foods – the ones only your closest people know about you. There were no silly shower games, just fun polls to learn about each other, like whose birthday was closest to my son's. A beautiful flower crown had been made for me. Surrounded by friends and family that I love and who love me. It was a perfect day, and an absolute change in seasons. Yet it was one many had been eagerly waiting to celebrate with me for years.

I knew I wouldn't be able to think on the spot, so I took the time to prepare a little thank you to those who attended. I wanted to thank them for their gifts, love and support through the past seven years.

"Thank you so much for coming today, I am so grateful for each of you. I never imagined myself in this situation. As I was going through and planning and preparing for what we may need for Anuwat, I teared up multiple times while imagining reading beautiful books to my son, playing with him, sharing meals, and snuggling with him on his bed. Praying that he will feel secure, loved, and cherished as he transitions into our family. That he will deeply feel that he has meant to be with us all along. We have been hoping and praying for Anuwat for over seven years. I have learned that some of the most special things in life take time, faith, and perseverance. In everything I've worked towards in my life, having Anuwat as my son tops the charts. Every moment of hoping, praying, and waiting has been worth it, and I haven't even met him yet. Thank you for sharing your time with me today and for your support and love along the way. For many, it's been a long road of navigating the ups and downs of this journey with me. I appreciate each and every one of you for the part you've played and the importance you hold in my life. My family and friendships are among the greatest blessings in my life and I love you all."

There's incredible potential shifting from the rigidity of clinging to our best-laid plans to holding them more loosely. *Shifting* plans is more of a *sifting* process. When we sift, we release the unnecessary elements and what remains is the treasure. The treasure we are meant to hold, where we are meant to be, who we are meant to be.

We don't plow or bulldoze our way through; the sifting process involves a character-stretching period that can't be sped through or launched in fast forward. I'm thankful for the change in my plans, and I'm grateful beyond words for them leading us to Pete.

Uncertainty remains, yet so does hope.

We discover that we can do hard things when we do hard things. Infertility is hard. Going through it, being in it, and experiencing it is hard. An incredible strength is elicited and revealed when we tune into it and acknowledge it. You are stronger than you think. This situation has been more challenging than I ever thought I could handle or go through. And yet, I went through it. You're going through it too. Moving one foot in front of the other, despite everything in your head telling you that you can't. Your circumstances are tough, but you are tougher. Strength doesn't mean powering through hard things at the expense of yourself. It might be a softening with the experience, a molding adjustment process, and quiet strength of overcoming. Strength is not always an outward display of mute emotions when times are tough, but the vulnerability of experiencing the pain, the hurt and the struggle. Working through it in the hopeful knowledge that the best is yet to come. Courage can only exist when fear or uncertainty is present; the uncertainty builds resilience when we hitch ourselves to courage.

Resiliency is "the capacity to recover from difficulties; toughness."[17] Resiliency requires self-compassion. Showing myself compassion, giving space for all of my imperfections, and treating myself kindly during these challenging times has helped to improve my resilience – my ability to recover from setbacks and difficulties. Tough times are the best teaching times. Understanding what I was saying to myself, how I was treating myself, and refining these responses to be those that I would share with a loved one helped soften this process. Expectations aren't perfection but progress when we are our own best friends. We are human and offer support in times of struggle, not judgment.

Wherever you are in this current season, your story isn't over yet. Your life doesn't have to be tied off in a bow before you live it. None of ours are. To be human is to suffer, love, learn, struggle, and grow. Lean into all of it. You are valuable, loved, and worthy. Your infertility does not define you, but it can refine you. Be gentle with yourself and your heart. Find the opportunity in the context of your reality.

Words of Wisdom From Those Who've Been There

When you know, you know. Those who have been through infertility understand this pain in a way that others can't. Here are some beautiful words of wisdom from people who have been there and get it. Excerpts from the online infertility survey revealed some incredible truths:

- This journey is incredibly difficult, and there will be sacrifices, but it is worth it no matter what outcome is meant for you.

- Find your support system, both inside and outside of your family.

- Distance yourself from the outcome. There is much to learn and appreciate along the journey.

- Buy comfortable pants; take a day off for yourself when needed.

- Give yourself permission to take as long as you need to mourn losses.

- Keep a flexible and realistic mindset.

- It's okay to feel sad for myself and happy for others; we can handle both.

- Take the time you need to focus on your relationship with your partner. Infertility isn't the end of a road but can begin a new path.

- There can be peace after infertility.

- Feel all of the feelings to help process them along the way. There are many.

- Let go. It's the hardest thing to do, especially initially, but it is far beyond your control. Cry more and be more open and willing to give yourself space and time to process. Don't try so hard.

- Be patient. Don't be obsessed with making babies. Take it one day at a time, and don't lose yourself in the process.

- You're going to be okay. Not being a mother is okay. You're not less of a woman for not having a child. If you want to be a parent, you will. Stop feeling like you're broken. Not having children doesn't mean you're not valuable. You are still worthy of love.

- You are not alone. It is okay to feel sad. To feel sorry for yourself. To be jealous. To be angry. But do not live in those feelings. Acknowledge them, and accept them. Remember that you are resilient.

- Be patient and have a listening ear for your husband – he's grieving too, and his anger is fear and grief. You will process differently – so much grace.

- You can't control this. No matter how many times you look at your calendars, it won't change anything. Enjoy life now, don't be so preoccupied about what you want your future to look like. You will have the family you were meant to have.

- This will likely be the most challenging journey you have ever gone on. Be brave, be strong and know your limits. It's okay to take breaks. It's okay to be sad, scared, angry, quiet, and loud. It's okay to be done. Just make sure that you do enough to have no regrets.

- Infertility is not your identity, and this journey will not last forever. Find support in others who have experienced infertility, and set boundaries for things like baby showers.

- Hard days will come, but it's okay to be carried, to ask for help, to let tears come quickly. It's okay to speak up for yourself and say when things hurt or make you uncomfortable.

YOUR INFERTILITY
LEGACY

Perhaps these terms seem odd together, infertility *and* legacy. Infertility isn't precisely what I think about when pondering legacy, either. What comes to mind when *you* think about legacy? Perhaps how you want others to feel when they think of you, the efforts you made towards making the world a better place, or the character traits that best describe you. When I think of the legacy of important people in history, or the valued people in my life that have passed, their resilience comes to mind.

What did they do when things *didn't* go as planned? We think of the times when the odds were stacked against them, and they put one foot in front of the other to move forward and keep fighting for what they believed in. When I think of the legacy of my late mother, I think of how she made me feel. I think of her giving spirit and sacrifice to love her family well, encouraging and building us up even when she was sick. On the hardest days, towards the end of her health struggles, she prioritized focus and attention on what mattered most to her: her family and her faith. She didn't feel sorry for herself. Or maybe she did for a time, but that didn't stick, and that's not what I remember. What lingers in her legacy is a life of loving others and prioritizing what meant the most, even when the going got tough.

Maybe legacy and infertility aren't clashing ideas after all, but an opportunity for clarifying this experience. There is an opportunity in the infertility journey to view your struggle in the context of a more incredible picture; your legacy of this battle. It's not a battle you chose to face, not a battle you'd wish anyone else to encounter. But it's here. You're in it. Keep going. This is tough, but you are tougher.

My dear friend Nicole Langman, MSW (author of *You Are Wanted – Reclaiming the Truth of Who You Are*), asked me a question recently that had me thinking. *What would you tell her if you were to speak to your five-year younger self?* It took me a few moments to process this question's simple yet complex depth. So much life has been lived in the past five years. For me, it boils down to a few key things:

Allow things to unfold.

Infertility requires action, and there is no way around it. In the actions taken, I would tell myself to leave space to let it unfold. Do what needs to be done, but don't try to hijack the situation and falsely claim more power over more than is possible. Create margin and leave breathing room for your story to come to be, as it's meant to. Clinging tighter, pushing harder, and controlling more increases the resistance and decreases joy.

Trust the process.

This challenge is not what anyone would choose, trust that this journey is yours and there is purpose in the process. Trust it.

Good can be experienced along with the hard.

Keep looking for the good while you're on the journey. It's not all hard and not all bad. Let them coexist.

Accept support from others.

Even the ones who don't understand. Help them know and let them know the best way to support you. Break the silence that so often encompasses the infertility journey.

Seasons change.

In the rough seasons, it's hard to see any way out. One thing is always certain, and that is change. It won't be like this forever. At some point, tides turn, and seasons change. You will not be *in* this struggle forever.

Good things are coming.

We traveled to Thailand in December 2020 and were quarantined for two weeks in a hotel in Bangkok, just eight minutes from the orphanage our son called home. A day after the quarantine was over, we met our perfect son, Pete, and our lives have never been the same. He is a dream come true – an absolute joy and delight. Our world was rocked most beautifully in the form of our two-and-a-half-year-old son. He is our missing puzzle piece, and we are blessed beyond measure. Life is hard, and life is good.

The concept of legacy in infertility offers a level of ownership of the experience. Our circumstances have us in this reality. Our ownership of this experience allows us to define the legacy we want to leave as we navigate it. Legacy is intentional, and it involves purposeful living. It doesn't subtract tough days or painful emotions. Instead, it honors the hard and the pain. It allows the hurt and the hope to dance together in the same room.

One day you will tell your story of this journey. What's the story you want to tell? Your hurt and your hope can co-exist. Make it count. We have one shot at this life. You are strong, you are resilient, you are valued and worthy. You are writing your infertility legacy story as we speak. I am cheering you on to your joy-filled future.

ABOUT THE AUTHOR

Karen Snow is a naturopathic doctor who is passionate about all aspects of improving the health of others. She loves supporting others on their health journeys for them to thrive. Along her family-building journey, she found herself experiencing infertility without a roadmap on how to navigate the complexities. The hope of offering support to others sharing this experience prompted the writing of this book.

She lives on a farm in rural Ontario with her husband Erik, son Pete, and their chocolate lab, Buddy.

Thank for you purchasing and reading my book. It was a joy to share our experience with you. This book project was difficult and took many years to complete. I hope that you found it valuable in your journey. Please consider leaving a review for this book online. Your support and feedback are greatly appreciated and will help others with their infertility journey.

References

1. Baikie KA, Wilhelm K. Emotional and physical health benefits of expressive writing. Advances in Psychiatric Treatment. 2005;11(5):338-346. doi:10.1192/apt.11.5.338

2. Brickman P, Campbell DT. Hedonic relativism and planning the good society. In: Appley MH, ed. Adaptation Level Theory: A Symposium. Academic Press; 1971:287-302. Cited by: Diener E, Lucas RE, Scollon CN. Beyond the hedonic treadmill: Revising the adaptation theory of well-being. American Psychologist. 2006;61(4):305-314.

3. Ben-Shahar T. Happier: Learn the Secrets To Daily Joy and Lasting Fulfillment. 1st ed. McGraw-Hill Education; 2007.

4. Phillips J. How coping with grief can affect your brain. Henry Ford Health Systems. Published June 4, 2018. https://www.henryford.com/blog/2018/06/how-coping-with-grief-can-affect-your-brain#

5. Brown B. Rising Strong. Random House; 2015.

6. Brown B quotes unnamed priest. 3 Ways to Recharge When You're Burned Out. Published online 2014.

https://www.oprah.com/inspiration/brene-brown-how-to-handle-burnout

7. Neff K. Self-Compassion: The Proven Power Of Being Kind To Yourself. William Morrow Paperbacks; 2015.

8. Holden R. Authentic Success: Essential Lessons and Practices From the World's Leading Coaching Program On Success Intelligence. Hay House; 2011.

9. Peoples D, Rovner Ferguson H. Experiencing Infertility: An Essential Resource. W W Norton; 2000.

10. EMD Serono. Ovidrel: PreFilled Syringe. Published online 2018. https://www.emdserono.com/us-en/pi/ovidrel-prefilled-syringe-pi.pdf

11. LR Knost. Little Hearts/Gentle Parenting Resources; 2016

12. Brown B. Atlas of the Heart; 2021

13. LearnVest. 10 Signs you're burning out – and what to do about it. Forbes. Published online April 1, 2013. https://www.forbes.com/sites/learnvest/2013/04/01/10-signs-youre-burning-out-and-what-to-do-about-it/?sh=50cc2fb3625b

14. Daigle L. Trust in You. Centricity; 2016.

15. Parker M. Adventure. Drom; 2016.

16. Adventure. In: Merriam-Webster Dictionary. Merriam-Webster; 2022. https://www.merriam-webster.com/dictionary/adventure#etymology

17. Resiliency. In: Oxford Dictionaries. Lexico Powered by Oxford; 2022. https://www.lexico.com/definition/resilience

18. Nagoski E, Nagoski A. Burnout: The Secret to Unlocking the Stress Cycle. Ballantine Books; 2019.

19. Gottman J, Silver N. The Seven Principles for Making Marriage Work: A Practical Guide from the Country's Foremost Relationship Expert. Harmony; 2015.

20. Morgan Cron I, Stabile S. The Road Back To You. Formatio; 2016.

Resources

- Self Compassion by Kristin Neff
- I Thought it was Just Me by Brené Brown
- Rising Strong by Brené Brown
- The Road Back to You by Ian Morgan Cron, Suzanne Stabile
- Burnout by Emily and Amelia Nakosky
- Conquering Infertility by Dr. Alice Domar
- For Those with Empty Arms: A Compassionate Voice for Those Experiencing Infertility Emily Harris Adams
- Mothers in Waiting: Healing and Hope for Those with Empty Arms by Crystal Bowman, Meghann Bowman
- Navigating Infertility: A tool to help guide you on your family building journey by Emily Day
- Infertility and PTSD: The Uncharted Storm by Joanna Flemons
- Unsung Lullabies: Understanding and Coping with Infertility by Janet Jaffe, Martha Ourieff Diamond, David J. Diamond
- The Infertility Survival Guide by Judith C. Daniluk
- Empty Womb, Aching Heart by Mario Schalesky

Karen would love to connect. You can find her online:

www.karensnow.ca
www.infertilitylies.com
www.facebook.com/DrKarenSnowND
www.instagram.com/karensnownd
www.instagram.com/infertilitylies

Made in United States
Troutdale, OR
02/19/2024

17798053R00135